A MEASURE OF LIGHT

Surviving sepsis and reclaiming my spirit

Kirsten Lavine

A Measure of Light
Surviving sepsis and reclaiming my spirit
by Kirsten Lavine

A catalogue card for this book is available from the British Library.

ISBN: 978-1-9998102-0-7

First published 2017

TJ INK
tjink.co.uk

Printed and bound by TJ International, Cornwall, UK

To Trevor, for his tireless support and dedication, and without whom none of this would be possible. And to everyone who helped towards making this book a reality – a very big thank you.

AUTHOR'S NOTE

All events detailed in this book are true and occurred pretty much as described, with small allowances and omissions made for the sake of clarity.

All characters in this book appear in their exact roles, but with the exception of my name and Trevor's, all names of people and places have been changed to protect their identities. Any names coinciding with true-life individuals and locations have occurred entirely by coincidence.

INTRODUCTION

'Oh hello!' said a bright-eyed nurse, gazing at me from the other end of the bed with surprise. 'I wondered what had happened to you!' I had wondered too. I had no idea who this nurse was, even once she had filled me in on our time together two weeks earlier. As she surmised, I had disappeared – both physically and mentally. And it was a long, long time before I came back again.

On 30 July 2015, I went into hospital for a basic day procedure called a hysteroscopy. Another nurse later told me that they perform twenty of these routine procedures a week, all without incident. I, on the other hand, ended up in intensive care in a coma for a week and a half and nearly died. This is my story of what happened, how I came back from another world and the lessons I have learned along the way.

The freakish turn of events I experienced has been the clearest demonstration of how sharply an unforeseen situation can crash into your world and bring death to your doorstep without warning. Having survived this catastrophe, my aims in writing this book are both to awaken people to the potential devastation of a life-threatening illness such as sepsis, but equally to empower individuals to take charge of their own recovery. So, while working in tandem with an appropriate medical treatment, is it important only to tread the path of healing that is right for you, and to continue to follow this path on your road to recovery thereafter.

This journey has been one of self-discovery and pain, of having the courage to stick to what you feel is right and to follow it through, even in the most alarming and adverse circumstances, and without losing the essence of who you are or what you believe in.

But this is also a story of love, loyalty, perseverance and hope, and of rediscovering and tasting the fragility of life and being grateful for the opportunity to heal again and become a part of its joy. It is a call to live life to your fullest, and to breathe and taste every moment as if it could very possibly be your last.

I have always considered myself to be a deeply spiritual person, though this entailed moving away from the organised religion of my upbringing in favour of a more alternative path of trying to live harmoniously and respectfully with people and my environment. I also elected to be a vegan over twenty years ago, and care passionately about nature and wildlife.

I suppose, given how unconventional my life has been in general, I perhaps should not have been so surprised that a rare foray into a routine medical procedure should have resulted in such a calamity. I have lived my life with a continual stream of uncertainty, ever since I left the bustling metropolis of Toronto, Canada where I grew up, in favour of a calmer, more old-fashioned style of life in England over twenty years ago.

During that time, I have lived in a number of places throughout the British Isles and abroad, which has resulted in a fairly patchy educational and work history. In between bouts of English language teaching and a variety of administrative roles, I managed to carve for myself a small niche in oral history, conducting interviews and compiling stories for various publications. As this work is always project based, it is therefore limited in longevity, and in between projects I have reverted to freelance teaching, editing, transcription and temporary admin roles.

In the midst of this constant state of flux, a relatively consistent factor in my life has been my one-time partner and still best friend, Trevor, a British music teacher raised in Northern Ireland, where we met. We've known each other for nearly fifteen years now, and still live together in the same house in England, where we've been for the past six years. Trevor has been the closest thing I've had to family in the UK. My actual family is in Canada, and consists primarily of an elderly mother (my father being deceased) and one older brother and his family. I Skype regularly with my mum and occasionally email my brother, and visit them once a year, usually in the summer. It would be fair to say that we're not very close, and Trevor has gone a long way towards filling the emotional void. He has been an unfailing support to me over the years, including his help in mitigating the sometimes uncertain circumstances of my chronic health condition.

It is this underlying disorder, called endometriosis, which brought me to undergo the hysteroscopy in the first place. This condition is starting to become better known, but many, like me, had never heard about it until I first embarked on this particular journey of investigation in 2010. Endometriosis can develop in females from any age after menstruation, but is especially common in women in their thirties and forties. The condition occurs when endometrial tissue grows abnormally outside of the womb and in other areas of the pelvis, and sometimes occurs in other parts of the body entirely. It can result in a myriad of symptoms, including heavy periods, problems with digestion and other types of pain.

Like many women, although I had probably suffered unknowingly for years with endometriosis, ironically, it wasn't any of its direct symptoms which led me to a diagnosis. Instead, many years ago, I started bleeding mid-cycle, which is not a normal state, and which has the potential to be an early sign of cancer. In 2009, when my father died of cancer – albeit a different kind – it heightened my concerns, and I decided I ought to determine the underlying cause of the bleeding.

After many consultations and tests, I agreed to undergo a laparoscopy and hysteroscopy in July 2010. The laparoscopy, or keyhole surgery, was to diagnose whether I had the suspected endometriosis, while the hysteroscopy was to ascertain the cause of the irregular bleeding. I underwent this procedure reluctantly and with some degree of fear, because I had never had any kind of surgery at all, nor very much to do with hospitals as a patient. The results of the laparoscopy showed that I had severe bilateral endometriosis. The hysteroscopy, which involves inserting a thin telescope into the womb through the cervix, had to be abandoned due to a blockage in my cervix, so any results were inconclusive.

This is where I had left it for years, countering any adverse effects of endometriosis with a healthy vegan diet and lifestyle, and an intuitive communication with my body. I was generally in good health overall and rarely became ill in any way. Unlike many other endometriosis sufferers, I didn't want to go down the road of taking hormones, which can cause equally negative symptoms, or to undergo several rounds of surgery to 'try and get rid of it'. Instead, I continued to handle the manageable symptoms and irregularities on my own. However, several years later I decided to revisit the situation. I was older now, in my forties (and the risk of certain types of cancer increases with age), and I was still bleeding irregularly, perhaps more than I had been before.

When I went for an initial consultation at the hospital, I said to a junior doctor, 'I suppose if it was cancer I wouldn't be alive to talk to you now,' to which she said nothing. I repeated this to the consultant, Mr Ellis, shortly after, and his reply to my assessment of not having cancer was, 'Not necessarily'. This alone was enough to scare me into investigating via another attempt at a hysteroscopy, which would be performed by him in a month's time, with biopsies taken and examined.

Working freelance gave me immeasurable degrees of flexibility, and I also blocked out the weekend after the surgery to recover. I'd been informed by Mr Ellis, and had read through the hospital literature about it being a fairly straightforward procedure and routinely performed, with the risks of any serious complications being very low. I overcame my fears and felt that it was best to have conclusive information as to the source of the bleeding. It was with this frame of mind that I entered hospital for the day surgery on Thursday 30 July 2015.

Trevor drove me to the gynaecological ward at 10 a.m. I was feeling reasonably sanguine about the whole affair. I'd just come back from a visit to Canada to see my family and was feeling healthy and well, having been immersed in sunshine and warmth for a few weeks. Having had the diagnostic laparoscopy, I felt I knew something of what to expect, and as such, entered Hawthorn Ward with a reasonably calm frame of mind.

After checking in with the receptionist, I was given a bed in a room with a few other women and waited until the anaesthetist came to talk with me, and then the surgeon, Mr Ellis, who summarily went through the consent form with me, which included an outline of the procedure and a checklist of potential risks.

I don't remember much after that except waking up, feeling woozy from the anaesthetic. At 4 p.m. I called Trevor and he came to the hospital. As mentioned, we are best friends now, but having been in a relationship for many years before, we agreed that he would effectively act as my partner or next of kin, to avoid any ambiguity about his presence on the ward or involvement in my care.

Trevor waited with me while I recovered, which included me vomiting twice from the remains of the anaesthetic, the same as I had done after the previous laparoscopy. Trevor noticed that I was hot and sweaty, but thought it was due to the paracetamol I'd been given and suggested I only be given ibuprofen. A doctor's visit established that the procedure had gone according to plan and that everything appeared to be fine. I later learned that the results from the biopsies were normal and that the irregular bleeding was attributed to my endometriosis. That afternoon I was assured that my post-operative state was normal, and that any cervical pain I was experiencing would have been caused by equipment used during the procedure.

At 7 p.m. I slowly got dressed to go home, and embarked on what I thought would amount to a few days of proper rest and recovery. I went straight to bed and tried to rest, as did Trevor. At 11 p.m. I started to feel pain in my upper abdomen – a place far from the site of my surgery, but I took some ibuprofen and tried to settle. I must have nodded off again, but at 4 a.m. I called Trevor into the room as I was awash with unbearable abdominal pain. I took more ibuprofen but nothing eased and I vomited it up. I should pause to say that I am not one of life's natural vomitters, so it would take ingesting a powerful substance or a serious situation for me to throw up.

Once Trevor saw me vomiting he called the hospital for advice. They told him to try paracetamol, and I berated myself for refusing to bring home the samples they offered because I generally did not get on with paracetamol. But Trevor duly drove out to an all-night ASDA and procured some. I took some paracetamol and after half an hour threw it up too. Trevor called the hospital again and they suggested I come in. I was in so much pain that it took a long time for me to get dressed.

We eventually made it into the car at about 6.30 a.m., just as the first light was dawning.

We arrived at Hawthorn Ward shortly thereafter and were asked to wait in the reception area. I could barely sit up and was in terrible pain. After an agonising hour, I was brought into an examination room and seen to by a nurse.

It's at this point my memories begin to get hazy. The next chapter, written by Trevor, offers a summary of events from that point onwards and over the next two weeks. My version of events, as I understood them to have occurred, appears in the following chapter.

PART 1

INTENSIVE CARE:
TREVOR'S STORY

Return to hospital

After an excruciating hour of waiting in the reception area of Hawthorn Ward that Friday morning, Kirsten was shown into an observation room. An intravenous drip was started but she was too ill to be properly examined. She was then taken to a bed on the ward and given Oramorph – a powerful morphine-based liquid painkiller, used regularly in hospital.

By noon, Kirsten seemed to be stabilising but still had considerable abdominal pain. The medical team were becoming perplexed. She was given an anti-spasmodic drug, which was the first thing to bring her relief. This suggested that the pain was being caused by some sort of bowel-related issue. She was taken via ambulance to the X-ray unit in the main building, and went again later for a CT scan and was given antibiotics. By the evening, Kirsten was still obviously in considerable pain, but she was now able to sit at rest in the bed. It was suggested that I go home and get some sleep.

Early the next morning, I arrived to find Kirsten looking very ill but slightly more rested than the previous day. She was seemingly returning to her normal self, asking for various things from home and for some fruit, so I popped round to the shops as per our usual Saturday morning routine, and felt a sense of normality returning.

When I returned from the shops, Kirsten was showing signs of wanting to go home but still looking very poorly. At around 10 a.m., several medics arrived on the scene to examine Kirsten, including a gynaecological consultant who introduced herself as Sandra, who worked closely with Mr Ellis, the surgeon who had performed the original surgery.

From Kirsten's symptoms that morning – very low blood pressure, coupled with an abnormally fast heart rate and mottled blue/grey skin – Sandra began to suspect that Kirsten was exhibiting some of the classic signs of having developed severe sepsis, a serious infection that required immediate treatment. This suspicion was confirmed shortly after, when a nurse came in and announced that Kirsten's white blood cell count had dropped further from the day before, which is a chief indicator of sepsis.

The energy of the scene changed immediately, and doctors and nurses started rushing in and out. Sandra began to talk about sending Kirsten to the intensive care unit (ICU) and conducting an exploratory laparoscopy to see what was going on. I could see Kirsten getting more and more agitated about all the fuss being made and I asked that they give her some time to rest, which they acceded to. Kirsten also urged me to go teach my ukulele group that afternoon, and sometime later texted me: 'Am moving to IC unit now for the next 24 hrs.'

When I returned to the hospital later that afternoon, I found Kirsten in the ICU in a room on her own, sitting in bed talking to a doctor. Her arms had been massacred by recent attempts at putting lines into her veins, which had become very faint as a result of her horribly low blood pressure.

However, she seemed to be feeling better, and asked me to fetch some of the grapes I had bought and was storing in a fridge in Hawthorn Ward. Kirsten was still adamant that she did not want further surgery. She was very cross that she had agreed to the original operation, and the last thing I remember her telling me was that she didn't want to die as a result of all this.

On returning to the ICU with the grapes, I was kept from seeing Kirsten. I didn't know where she was or what was happening with her. I was surprised to be told that she'd been taken to theatre. I later discovered that Kirsten had developed worse abdominal pain, and Sandra had decided to perform a laparoscopic washout to ensure that Kirsten didn't have a perforated bowel, and to try and identify the source of the sepsis, the progress of which was becoming increasingly severe.

I was encouraged to go home for a while, so I did, and freshened up for the 24 hours to come, which I knew would be crucial to Kirsten. As it was Saturday, the day she normally Skyped with her mum in Canada, she had asked me to contact her, but with a much-reduced version of what was going on. Although her elderly mother knew about the original surgery, Kirsten didn't want to communicate any of the seriousness of how the situation had progressed. So I emailed her mum and told her that her daughter was staying on in hospital with an infection. I also made a *'Get Better Kirsten'* sign and photographed it with her cuddly animals holding it up, ready to show her when she came round.

The darkest night

Later that evening I returned to the ICU. I was asked to wait for quite a while in the 'Quiet Room'. Scott, a consultant anaesthetist, eventually came in to speak to me. He told me that Kirsten was critically ill and might not make it, but he assured me that he and his team would do everything they could for her. He explained that sepsis is a life-threatening condition, where the body reacts abnormally to an infection by attacking its own tissues and organs. With Kirsten's blood pressure continuing to fall, she had entered the final and potentially fatal stage of 'septic shock', which can often lead to multiple organ failure and death.

He suggested that I begin to keep a diary, because if Kirsten did pull through, it was going to be a long process, and it would be good for her to have a record of all the time she would have lost. I'm not sure I could really cope with all that I was hearing, but I thought the best thing I could do was to go deep within myself and try to reach Kirsten from within.

At 11.30 p.m. I was invited into the room, and was dismayed to discover Kirsten lying under thin, grey blankets, amidst an array of tubes and pipes and machines. She had been put in a medically-induced coma and intubated, which entailed breathing through a tube attached to a ventilator.

The main nurse responsible for Kirsten was a gentle girl called Imogen, who we had met the previous afternoon. Imogen explained all the various monitors and medical paraphernalia to me, but encouraged me to fix my attention on Kirsten and not to become engrossed by the equipment. Kirsten had also been fitted with a tube which allowed liquids to be passed directly into her stomach. As I let Imogen know that Kirsten was a strict vegan (and it turned out Imogen was a vegan too), Kirsten was given a soya feed instead of cow's milk.

Despite the dire situation Kirsten was going through, the ICU staff did a very good job of making her look as if she were comfortable and clean and on the road back to health. She had her hair tied back and was very well presented, and other than having oedema, a condition which resulted in a very bloated appearance in her face and hands from all the excess fluid given to her, Kirsten looked remarkably normal, and in no way like someone who was in danger of dying at any moment.

I was given a comfortable chair to sit on next to Kirsten's bed. I felt that I was being allowed to be there because I was a vital link for Kirsten with her normal life within this totally alien environment. As such, I decided to pretty much meditate as much as I could, and only speak whenever I was spoken to.

At 12.30 a.m. I told the duty nurse that I was planning on sitting quietly with Kirsten throughout the night while she slept until the morning. I really felt that I wanted to be there at the moment when Kirsten regained consciousness. What I didn't realise was that there would be an army of people in and out all night. With the escalation of the infection to septic shock, Kirsten's blood pressure had become alarmingly low, which was the main issue that could cause her to die. As such, throughout the night the team were pumping Kirsten with a steady stream of fluids and the hormone noradrenaline, in the hope that her body would stabilise. The main doctor in charge, a serious and intense man, was checking Kirsten's blood pressure every half hour and telling Imogen to give Kirsten more fluid because her blood pressure wasn't rising out of the immediate danger zone.

It was 6.30 a.m. before Kirsten's blood pressure was eventually brought to a stable level. I didn't want to leave, as I still believed that she would come round, and I wanted to be there to show her the picture of the animals I had made for her. Little did I know that this was merely the start of a long and protracted medically-induced coma, out of which Kirsten would be lucky to emerge alive.

The battle begins

Later that morning, Scott, the consultant anaesthetist, gave me a rundown of the situation. He repeated exactly how ill Kirsten was and warned me that this would be a very long process. He also reiterated the theory that the pressurised water used in Kirsten's hysteroscopy had led to blocked material in her uterus – which contained E. coli bacteria – being pushed out and into her body cavity, where it had become a 'septic shower' in her body and had started to infect Kirsten's entire abdominal area.

They were keeping her in a medically-induced coma so that her body could stabilise while they treated the infection.

Scott was accompanied by another doctor, who turned out to be Mr Ellis, the gynaecologist who had carried out the hysteroscopy. Ellis said the next few weeks would be critical, and depending on how certain inflammatory markers responded to treatment, they would review the situation in terms of any additional surgery that might be required.

Ellis asked how I was coping, and Scott, being equally concerned with my health, suggested that I head on home and get some rest. I went home, had lunch, showered and changed, and returned that afternoon. The nurses asked me to give them some time to tend to Kirsten, so I sat on the chair in the corridor and looked into the sky, and noticed the sunlight shining on the clouds. When the medical team allowed me to return, I sat next to Kirsten until they sent me home around midnight, with orders to get lots of rest.

I passed most of Monday and Tuesday sitting with Kirsten as much as I could. She remained in a medically-induced coma, and for an hour or two in the mornings, was brought round by way of the sedation being switched off. The medical team monitored her progress in combatting the infection, which was being treated mainly with antibiotics. A large easel in the room propped up Kirsten's medical chart, which listed every iota of medication and fluid passing in and out of her, all of which were painstakingly recorded and cross-referenced with each new nurse arriving on shift.

Kirsten's ability to absorb food was also very poor, another aspect being closely monitored. She was still being given a soya feed, and this was written up on a large whiteboard at the back of the room, along with other personal details about Kirsten, including her love of Ludovico Einaudi's piano music, which was obtained from the internet and played continuously, until I began to bring these CDs from home.

It was fortunate that it was summer and I had very few teaching commitments, so I was able to be at the hospital most of the day, with one or two music lessons to teach at home in the evenings. I was told visiting hours were from 10 a.m., so my routine became calling first thing in the morning to check with the night nurse, and aiming to arrive at 10 a.m. I sometimes had to wait while they were doing something with Kirsten, but generally nobody questioned my being there the whole day. Once I realised Kirsten wasn't going to be coming home with me any time soon, I stopped coming by car, as parking at the hospital was a nightmare. We lived nearby, so I could cycle instead and lock my bike very close to the ICU.

Tuesday evening after my flute lesson, I decided it would be a good idea to check Kirsten's emails to see if any of her friends had contacted her over the past few days and were waiting to hear from her. I wrote to each of them, mostly in general and optimistic terms, and promised to keep in touch. At least since Kirsten hadn't yet resumed her freelance work since returning from Canada, there weren't any work matters that required any immediate attention.

I must admit that I began to wonder if Kirsten would ever regain full consciousness. The fear was in me that perhaps something which happened during her time in the ICU would mean she would never be the same again. I decided to put this issue to the back of my mind, and put all energy into helping Kirsten get strong again.

On Wednesday morning, Kirsten's fourth day in intensive care, Justin, the consultant anaesthetist on duty, told me they had decided to proceed with another surgical washout conducted by Sandra. This was firstly to ensure that Kirsten didn't have a perforated bowel, but also to try and clear some of the gritty-looking fluid that had been flowing through the drainage tubes fitted to her abdomen. Kirsten went into her third trip to theatre and came out a couple of hours later.

As I sat with Kirsten, who was off sedation, she kept waving her arms around randomly. Every time she became aware of the tube down her throat she became very distressed, so I tried to reassure her that all the equipment she was encountering was doing a great job of making her better.

But as Kirsten was not showing any real signs of fighting the infection, and the medical team seemed to be giving me information only on a need-to-know basis, I began to imagine the worst. All sorts of thoughts were going through my mind about the many things that can lead to brain damage when someone is in such a vulnerable situation and dependent on IV fluids, in addition to having E. coli in the bloodstream.

The main strategy for quelling this infection was a regular administration of the antibiotic Tazocin several times a day. I only discovered much later that one of the main obstacles to Kirsten's recovery was that the particular strain of E. coli she had was resistant to most antibiotics normally used to combat this type of infection, so the Tazocin was limited in its effectiveness.

Extubation attempts

Later that morning, the team had decided to go for an extubation – the removal of the breathing tube, which would free Kirsten of the need for the ventilator and enable her to breathe on her own. The tube is usually kept in for as long as a patient needs help breathing while unconscious.

Extubation carries with it many considerations. If you take the tube out too soon, the patient may not be able to breathe, but leaving it in prolongs the process of sedation, weakening the patient further and opening them up to other problems like chest infections. If the person can breathe independently, they can eat and be more active, all of which better equips the body to fight an infection.

I was told by the doctors that there were certain criteria that needed to be met before they were willing to attempt an extubation, mainly that once the sedation had been switched off, Kirsten had to demonstrate a certain amount of physical strength and mental cognition.

That Wednesday morning, after about an hour of being free from sedation, Kirsten was still very drowsy, and waving her arms and legs like a baby. She was showing few signs of facial recognition and was not responding to verbal commands. 'Kirsten, squeeze my hand Kirsten, squeeze my hand...' She did squeeze my hand, but very much in her own time and seemingly not as a response. After about two hours of this, the nurse on duty suggested that it was getting too late to attempt an extubation, so they were going to put her back into sedation.

I sat with Kirsten, wondering if she would ever come round again, and looked on helplessly while she drifted back off to sleep on a high level of the sedative propofol. Then, as it was evening, I needed to head home to teach my flute student.

The next morning, Thursday, I found what seemed to be a more relaxed Kirsten. She'd had her sedation turned off for about thirty minutes, and for the first time seemed quite at peace and childlike. She was swinging her feet around and seemed to have come to terms with the breathing tube. I decided to see what Kirsten would do if confronted with Chubb Chubb, a big, plush snowy owl and one of her favourites, in the hope that seeing him would help bring her back to the level of wakefulness the doctors were requiring in order to take out the tube. The nurse put on a relaxing Einaudi piano CD and I produced the Chubb…to no effect! To be honest, a part of me felt better about some of the positively non-committal responses that I had been receiving from Kirsten, because if she didn't respond to Chubb Chubb, then there wasn't much hope for me!

Despite this lack of lucidity, when Justin, the consultant anaesthetist came round mid-morning, he decided to try for an extubation. I waited for an hour in the corridor, only for Justin to reappear to tell me that they'd had to put the tube back in again, because of the rapid loss of oxygen in Kirsten's bloodstream due to a too-weak breathing response from her. In other words – she was not strong enough to breathe on her own. Despite this seeming lack of progress, I still felt deeply that something had changed from the day before and Kirsten had turned a corner. I was only later to discover that this was most likely due to the fact that Kirsten had been given a new antibiotic the day before, meropenem, which proved to be the first one which had any real effectiveness in combatting the infection.

Tracheotomy

After the failed extubation, Justin presented me with a very tough dilemma. He strongly suggested giving Kirsten a tracheotomy – an incision in the windpipe. With a ventilation tube placed directly into her throat, Kirsten would be able to be conscious, move more freely and to build up her overall strength.

But as he spoke, something in me just could not accept that this was the best line of action to take. I knew how distressed Kirsten would be about having a permanent and visible scar on her neck. She often expressed to me how upset she was at the laparoscopy scar on her tummy button that, after four years, was only beginning to heal, and I felt as though she would not want to give her consent for this.

But in resisting this procedure, I was exposing her to extreme discomfort, a possible chest infection, and forcing her to experience a ventilation tube that was designed for an unconscious patient and not a conscious person. I was also giving the medical team an extremely difficult situation to have to deal with. But still I resisted, as I knew in my heart that this was not what Kirsten would have wanted. I was under a lot of pressure, and was amazed that while I was refusing to let them proceed via the tracheotomy route, that they were abiding by my wishes.

That afternoon I saw Stuart, a very kind nurse. He was very understanding about my reluctance to allow a tracheotomy, yet he gently pointed out the benefits of doing this, as Kirsten would be free to interact with the world in a natural way. I asked Stuart how common the tracheotomy route was and he said that it was very common, suggesting that we were going against the flow, and that a patient being linked to a respirator, while under relatively low levels of sedation, was not the usual way of things.

Later that afternoon Kirsten, in a semi-conscious state, was swinging her leg again over the side of the bed and exploring her arterial lines with her arms. By refusing the tracheotomy, I had basically volunteered to spend the days keeping her from yanking out her life lines. With no idea if this option would work, I grabbed hold of Kirsten's arms whenever it looked as if she was about to pull something out. But for the first time in a week, I managed to see Kirsten drift off into a peaceful sleep, and for that alone, what I had done had been worth it. It was just a question of keeping in there and hoping that she could get strong enough to reach the next stage on her own steam.

Lumbar puncture

The next morning, Friday, Justin told me there were positive signs, in that Kirsten had an increasingly healthy white blood cell count and had started to absorb nutrition once more. However, after six days in the ICU, Kirsten's rate of recovery was still slower than they were hoping.

It also became clear that the doctors shared my concerns for Kirsten's lack of higher mental processes, as Gavin, another consultant anaesthetist, came to me and asked for permission to run a CT scan of Kirsten's head and to carry out a lumbar puncture test. This entailed introducing a small needle into the base of Kirsten's spine, extracting spinal fluid, and checking it for impurities to see if any of the infection had managed to reach Kirsten's brain cavity.

I asked Gavin about the risks involved in the process, and he told me that there was a 1 in 60,000 chance that problems might arise from the procedure itself – considerably better odds than in the original hysteroscopy – so I decided that this would probably be a good thing to do and gave my consent.

I had an intuitive sense that Kirsten's state was more positive than his diagnosis, and suggested as much, drawing attention to the much more rested state that she had managed to achieve over the past couple of days. He said that he really hoped that I was right, but wanted to run the tests to be sure.

It was a long wait for the CT scan to be done, as Kirsten's appointment kept getting delayed in light of other emergencies which arose. When she was finally taken later in the afternoon, I resumed my seat in the corridor. As I waited for her to return, I thought about how this was probably the longest time in Kirsten's life that she had been away from being with the birds and the trees and sunlight. How I longed to be able to be with her as she used to be once more, out in nature, far away from the scientifically-controlled medical environment she had been swallowed by.

I began to reflect on all the little ways in which she had enriched my life – the joy of unfolding in the moment with her, walking in the woods, or along the river, or simply standing in the back garden under the rose arch. Or just going shopping at Sainsbury's, or seeing her cooking her lovely food in our tiny kitchen, or cycling off to meet one of her friends in the light rain, or learning Italian, or making the tea for our recorder group and sharing her thoughts on making music.

When Kirsten was brought back and looking settled, I got talking with one of the nurses and told her that I was able to see how the core of Kirsten had returned, a person with a very wonderful childlike nature, who found delight in the simplicity of the moment.

That night, I called Kirsten's mum in Canada. Having been nearly a week with few signs of a return to consciousness, I felt that I had respected Kirsten's wish for her mum not to be disturbed by these events long enough, and that it was now time to look at certain aspects of her state together. Her mum was quite taken aback in hearing that Kirsten had been in the ICU on ventilation, yet she remained calm and thanked me for letting her know. I was surprised at her reaction to all that I was telling her, to the extent that I'm not sure if it really sank in. I promised to keep her informed of any developments in Kirsten's situation. One thing that touched me deeply was when she said how pleased she was that Kirsten had me as a friend.

I wasn't sure how I felt at that stage. Something told me that Kirsten was by no means out of the woods. The only cure for this was to think only about the situation at hand, and not to dwell on any projected expectations of improvement.

Pelvic clearance surgery

The next morning, Saturday, I awoke at 8 a.m., having slept through the alarm. Immediately, I realised to my horror that I had missed the night nurse, so would not get a first-hand account of how Kirsten had been in the night – ah! I'd been up late the night before trying to get information on septic shock and had simply not heard the alarm. It's incredible to think that in the UK alone, 44,000 people a year die from sepsis. It was also still difficult for me to believe that Kirsten had contracted such a deadly disease from such a routine surgical procedure.

While I felt that Kirsten had turned a corner, I was still very wary of what the findings would be from the lumbar puncture and the CT scan. In the meantime, I got through to a nurse called Amy and was told some very encouraging news – Kirsten was showing signs of purposeful movement, as she was squeezing Amy's hand.

When I arrived at the hospital, and was eventually allowed in, I found Kirsten sitting upright in bed, awake, looking very puzzled and even annoyed. She had been without sedation for a while, and for the first time was showing real signs of recognition of her situation. She was indeed squeezing hands at command, and I asked her if she could hear the Einaudi music playing. From her facial expression she might have come out with something like: 'Of course I can hear the music but I don't really want to be in this situation!' So she was better, but not better enough for her liking.

Kirsten looked strangely healthy, if a little bloated from the oedema, with her hands, feet and face being much bigger than normal. Yet she had a good colour, and her eyes, which had been disturbingly distant and unfocused, took on more and more of a look that was filled with life and light. I also later learned that the lumbar puncture test had come back clear, free of any worrying signs.

At midday, Mr Ellis came to speak to me, and suggested that from the medical point of view, Kirsten was making slow but sure progress in the right direction, but that they were concerned with certain inflammatory markers that were on the rise, like the C-reactive protein (CRP), with normal being a measurement of 7, while Kirsten's CRP was still over 300. He told me that he hoped that this would settle down in time, and that she would be able to recover on her own.

However, he had in mind the option of 'pelvic clearance' surgery, which entailed the removal of the uterus, ovaries and fallopian tubes, which might be needed if Kirsten did not significantly improve. Despite the washout operations, there were still reservoirs of infected liquid deep in her pelvis that he thought could only be successfully addressed by this major abdominal surgery. I told him that if any further surgery were needed, then I would prefer it if Kirsten herself were in a situation to join in the decision process. Gavin later shared Ellis's views but expressed them with a greater sense of urgency. He suggested that unless this pelvic clearance surgery was undertaken imminently, Kirsten might slip back into a much worse state that would make her too weak to fight off the disease, and too weak to undertake any necessary surgery at a later stage.

That night I awoke at 3 a.m. with various thoughts going through my mind. One was the strange way in which Kirsten was breathing with the ventilator. There was part of me which felt that there was something in Kirsten thinking 'this is weird', and she was not fighting back but merely accepting the situation. I could imagine a scenario where Kirsten felt overwhelmed by the weirdness, and reached a point where letting go was more attractive than fighting to return.

It's very sad, but the day before I was trying to share my fears with a nurse, and she said: 'But she has you...' I realised now that if this was all she had, then it was simply not good enough. If Kirsten was to survive she needed to find and connect with her own energy, and if she couldn't do this then I needed to have the strength to let go.

A waiting game

At 7 a.m. the next morning, I called and asked how Kirsten had been in the night, and was told that she had been stable and was showing more signs of awareness, opening her eyes and exploring with her hands. She had also been squeezing hands on command. When I arrived that Sunday morning, Kirsten seemed quite alert and was making eye contact with Amy, the nurse. Amy was reading to her from a book about a cat, and it seemed as though the communication between them was much more full and grounded. However, Amy had just given Kirsten another sedative to ease her discomfort, and I could see that Kirsten was beginning to slip away again. But while I was holding her hand, I really felt a connection there that had not been there before, and that perhaps this was the first time she had recognised me.

Later in the morning, Gavin came round and told me that he was aware of my concerns over the tracheotomy. I repeated my deep conviction that I could not imagine Kirsten giving consent to such a move, and he reassured me that everything possible would be done to avoid this. Kirsten's breathing was remaining stable and she was holding out against the infection, so all being well they were going to try to extubate her again the next day.

That morning, a light-hearted incident occurred when a new nurse turned to me and asked: 'Are you Kirsten's dad?' I replied: 'Believe me, at the moment I feel like her granddad!' Laughingly, she said, 'Oh, so sorry. It's just that Kirsten looks so young!' The poor nurse doesn't know how much she cheered me up.

I spent much of the day holding Kirsten's hand and reassuring her when she coughed. Although I had only a few signs to go on, I felt that things were going in the right direction. I felt fortunate that I was able to stay calm for Kirsten, which is just what she needed at this time. She did very well overall, and hopefully would be strong enough for another attempt at extubation the next day.

Further struggles

The next morning, Monday 10 August, my 7 a.m. call to the nurse let me know that Kirsten was doing well and needed sedation throughout the night as she was being a little 'fighty', which was just what I wanted to hear.

At 10.15 a.m., I was allowed in and found Kirsten fast asleep. It was noon when Kirsten slowly came round, followed by the arrival of Mr Ellis and Sandra. Ellis told Kirsten that they were going ahead with their plan for extubation and asked her to nod if she understood, which she did. Despite this initial plan, Kirsten had to demonstrate that she was mentally capable of taking command of her situation and having the strength to do so. She had started to interact somewhat with people, which was a very good sign, but she needed to be able to raise her arms on command and she wasn't showing much evidence of being interested in doing this. The obvious result: no extubation that day. This gave everyone a problem – how is Kirsten to breathe?

I kept expecting them to come up with a reason why they had to perform an emergency tracheotomy.

I still felt terrible and anxious, that in refusing to let the team give Kirsten a tracheotomy, I may have been jeopardising Kirsten's return to health, forcing her to endure days of what can only be described as torture. I may also have been giving the medical team an altogether more taxing time in caring for Kirsten than they should have had.

The day before, I had spoken frankly with Amy about how I'd been trying to cope with the situation, witnessing what I was seeing Kirsten going through. I was also feeling very confused and full of self-doubt about the tracheotomy issue. Amy told me we can only do what we think is right, and it was not a good idea to question it too much. I thanked her for her professionalism and humanity.

That night I managed to stick it out until 9.40 p.m., then the powers that be very persuasively told me that I would not be allowed to stay on the ward overnight. I tried to explain how the situation was unusual, in that the doctors wanted to give Kirsten a tracheotomy but she did not want this, so I had agreed to stay and prevent her from pulling things out of herself.

This argument was met with the assurance that Kirsten would have a nurse with her all night, who was trained to sit with patients and make sure they came to no harm. It was time for me to leave and I expressed my thanks to everyone. When I got home, a nurse rang me to comfort me with the news that Kirsten was now sedated and sleepy.

Now that I had been forcibly removed from her side, she was basically all on her own. I had no idea what they were getting up to in the night. I was being kept from where I need to be, with Kirsten. I guessed that if she managed to yank out something they considered vital to their plan of care, then they would act. There had been talk of restraints being used...it just gets worse and worse. My worst fears were confirmed when, at 7 a.m. the next morning, I got through to the night nurse who told me that Kirsten had to be restrained with her arms tied to the bed to stop her from pulling her tubes out. The main problem was that Kirsten now needed two nurses, one to carry out the general monitoring and the other to prevent Kirsten from hurting herself.

Freed at last

Full of concern, I arrived at the ICU at 8.30am that Tuesday morning. I discovered the reception area deserted, so I phoned Kirsten's room and got through to an Irish nurse called Claire, who let me in. Kirsten was calm and lucid, and seemed to have been listening to Claire and nodding. I immediately knew that with Claire's sensitivity and focus, she had managed to reach Kirsten's intelligence and to communicate to her the seriousness of her situation and how vital it was for her to relax and not to try to fight her way out. At that moment, I knew that Kirsten was going to make it through this terrible challenge of being fully awake burdened with a tube designed for the unconscious. We spent a pleasant morning with me chatting with Claire and listening to classical music. Kirsten was obviously much better and was lifting her arms and coughing in response to being asked to.

At about 10 a.m., the anaesthetist, Scott came to pay Kirsten a visit: 'That tube needs to come out.' An hour later a party of doctors, including Gavin, arrived to make the decision. It was obvious that Kirsten was better, but was she better enough? Gavin decided to give it a go, and to be ready to re-intubate with enough time for her to settle should the need arise.

Kirsten looked non-committal, but through engaging people with eye contact, made them realise that she understood what they were saying to her.

I was asked to give them some space, so I went to get a coffee and eat my lunch. It was a lovely day and I could see the sun was shining outside. I had no idea whether or not Kirsten was going to make it through this second round of extubation, but in my heart I felt very much at peace about the whole situation.

When I returned, I discovered Kirsten back in the land of the living with no tube! Just an oxygen mask to help her through the next while. I was so relieved to see her freed from all that machinery. Kirsten started to try to talk, but it took her a long time to find her voice. Claire was great with Kirsten, especially when it came to drinking. Kirsten wanted lots of water but was curbed by Claire, who wanted to avoid complications post-extubation, since Kirsten's throat might have been too weak for her to be able to swallow liquids.

As the afternoon wore on, Kirsten was finding her voice more and more, and speaking in a rasping whisper. The message she was giving me was, 'Enough, I want to go home!' I still didn't think that she was 100 per cent lucid, but it was enough for her to avoid a huge hole in her throat. Having come this far today, I very much doubted if she would need to go back to that, but insisting on going home...?

We would see what the next while would bring – hopefully more control over her breathing, fewer signs of internal infection, fewer sources of pain and a lot more overall strength. Kirsten eventually said to me: 'I don't know what you expect,' as in, how you expect me to behave, to which I said, 'I expect nothing other than to see you get better...' which is the absolute truth.

By the evening Kirsten was more and more aware of her situation, and showing the first signs of interest in her life outside of her immediate illness, as she listened to me read the email messages her friends had written over the past ten days. She also confessed to Claire that she was a little confused. Claire was able to explain to her in very clear language just why she might be feeling confused, in light of all that she had just lived through.

We were lucky to have had Claire that day, as she had that mixture of sensitivity, professionalism and discipline that was perfect for Kirsten's most important day of the weaning process from ventilation to breathing on her own. I thanked Claire for her excellent job and wished Kirsten a peaceful night.

When I got home, I spoke to Kirsten's mum. I promised to keep her posted in the weeks to come and said I felt confident Kirsten would soon be able to speak to her directly. I had emailed her brother a few days before to update him. He offered his support and advice on dealing with some of the medical issues, and thanked me for being there for Kirsten.

The need to feed

The next morning, I got through to a very agitated nurse who told me that Kirsten had had a very unsettled night, during which she had tried to climb out of bed a few times, insisting that she be allowed to sit in the large chair in the room.

I arrived just after 10 a.m. Kirsten was looking very weak and had an oxygen facial mask strapped to her face to help her breathe. I found a new nurse looking after her – a large, young man who, it turned out, had been there overnight to prevent her from climbing out of the bed! Kirsten was clearly confused and angry and didn't want to stay in hospital, yet at this stage was a long way from being able to do anything about it.

Stuart the nurse arrived and told me that the physiotherapist was coming round to assess whether Kirsten was strong enough to sit in a chair, the one Kirsten had been insisting on being allowed to sit in. He also told me that Kirsten was having trouble swallowing after being on a ventilator so long, and to prevent her from becoming even more undernourished, the plan was to continue with a soya feed being pumped directly into her stomach. A dietician came and spoke to myself and Kirsten about this, as well as discussing the prospect of replacing the existing nasogastric (NG) tube with a longer nasojejunal (NJ) tube, in the hope that this would improve Kirsten's absorption levels, particularly of protein.

She also proposed giving Kirsten a regular intake of a nutritionally-rich (non-vegan) juice called Fortisip. I suggested that perhaps I could source a vegan version instead. I went off to our local health food shop and bought a load of protein drinks and soya yogurt, in the hope that Kirsten would like them enough to take them. I returned later that afternoon to find Kirsten sitting in the chair. She had been hoisted in it while I was out shopping. I set her up with soya yogurt, protein drinks and grape juice.

At 6 p.m., a young doctor appeared and announced that Kirsten had developed a form of candida, which they felt was important to treat with anti-fungal agents, which they duly applied. An hour later came the brightest aspect of the day – Kirsten tucked into soya yogurt and looked like she really was enjoying it.

The next day, Thursday, at lunchtime, two technicians wheeled in a scanning device, and wanted to remove Kirsten's NG tube and replace it with an NJ tube in the other nostril. Kirsten objected vehemently. She was becoming increasingly aware of all the lines she was connected to, and felt that this new tube would be even more painful than the one she already had.

It was around the time that they were serving meals, so I suggested that we try Kirsten with the old-fashioned method of eating. The nutritionists left, deciding to leave the task of fitting the tube until after lunch, though strangely, they never returned. It had been a week and a half since Kirsten had eaten properly, and had they known that the Asian noodles served for lunch gave her terrible wind, they might have come back, but we were already on course to launch a different plan.

In the meantime, Kirsten had asked me to fetch her laptop in the hope that she could go online and contact some of her family and friends for the first time since being admitted to hospital. While I was setting up the computer, Kirsten was busy pulling out her NG tube, becoming fed up with this alien object up her nose. There was nothing I could do – it was out in a flash. The nurse was quite pleased about this though, as it gave her an excuse to ask the nutritionists to put in the new NJ tube, though this was something that simply wasn't going to happen.

Instead, Kirsten and I discussed what foods we could get that would satisfy the level of nutritional intake that the medics were strongly suggesting she needed. I was sent off to fetch all sorts of foods that belonged to Kirsten's world, such as oatcakes, almond butter and spirulina. Kirsten was going to feed herself back to health, whatever it would take.

At 5.30 p.m., Mr Ellis arrived to see Kirsten sitting up in the chair, eating blueberries and soya yogurt and typing on her computer. He was very pleased to see how well Kirsten was looking, and stopped by the medical chart to check on the inflammatory markers. As he did so, Kirsten leaned over to me and made a wry comment, expressing her distress at coming face-to-face with the man who she felt was responsible for her landing in the ICU in the first place.

An hour later, Gavin appeared on his evening rounds. He saw Kirsten sitting up, using her computer and eating blueberries, some of which he was kicking around with his feet, as they had cascaded onto the floor, and which caused his normal downcast demeanour to lift into an unintentional smile. In spite of this moment of levity, Gavin was openly pessimistic about Kirsten's prognosis. He told her that he believed her to be one of the sickest patients in the hospital and that she needed to eat well in order to build up her strength to get better, or she might start to fall back into illness.

The next morning, Friday 14 August, the dietician returned to check on Kirsten's progress. I showed her the protein drinks and other foods I had bought. She seemed impressed with how well-informed we were in terms of understanding dietary needs, and agreed to delay the NJ tube's insertion, following a review of the situation when she returned on Monday. This effectively gave us the weekend to prove to the medical team that we could meet all that was expected in terms of nutrition. I was sent off to town with a shopping list, which included various things such as barley grass, almond butter, coconut oil, pea protein powder and kale.

The plan was for me to make up smoothies at home of soya or rice milk, spirulina and protein supplements during the day, and to make meals of lentils, beans and grains for the evening. I realised that the medical team were being very patient and understanding in giving me this chance, but for how long? Kirsten and I had to make this work.

Pelvic surgery resurfaces

Later on, as I was getting into the car with all of my shopping, my phone rang. It was Kirsten, who had just been visited by Mr Ellis. She was in a panic and wanted me to return as soon as possible. According to Kirsten, Ellis was returning after lunch with Sandra to discuss major abdominal surgery. Kirsten informed him that she wished to talk about this issue only when I was present. I threw the shopping into the car and was on my way!

When I arrived at the room, I found Kirsten sitting in the chair, very concerned about what Ellis and Sandra were going to say to her. By the time they arrived, Kirsten had made it perfectly clear to me that she wanted no more major surgical procedures. I decided to defend Kirsten's position, as I felt that this was the right way forward for her, and the best way to return her back over the line she had crossed from holistic health to modern scientific medicine.

While both doctors were positive about the 'downward trend of the inflammatory markers', which meant that Kirsten wasn't getting any worse, fundamentally they were there to try to persuade Kirsten to agree to the removal of her ovaries, fallopian tubes and enlarged uterus, in order to gain access to the last remaining reservoirs of infected fluid that were holding back Kirsten's recovery.

I tried to make it quite clear that a better line of action by far would be to explore every possible medical avenue towards Kirsten's recovery, before contemplating such drastic measures as a 'pelvic clearance'. They were both somewhat taken aback by our joint stand on the issue, but they seemed willing to respect our views – for the time being.

End of the ICU in sight

The next morning, Saturday, was warm and sunny, and there seemed to be an optimistic mood on the ICU. A new nurse was with Kirsten when I came in who was helping her walk to the loo, a curtained-off area five feet from her bed.

The morning rounds brought a new consultant, Dr Adams, a tall, thin man, full of quiet confidence. He gave a medical assessment of where Kirsten was after two weeks in the ICU. He reiterated the need for her to build up her strength by eating properly, but he was concerned that the antibiotics alone weren't proving effective enough to clear the infection. He acknowledged Kirsten's reluctance to undergo pelvic surgery, but held concerns that should she deteriorate further and then opt for the surgery, then she could find it much harder to recover, if she did at all. However, he had been looking at the CT scans of Kirsten's abdominal region and was enquiring into the possibility of a drainage procedure assisted by radiographic technology, something which sounded very high tech.

At this point Kirsten put forward her case, namely that she wanted to go home! I interrupted and tried to make Kirsten realise that she was waging a war with the E. coli infection and needed to be in hospital, so that she could keep taking the antibiotics to stop the pathogen completely engulfing her body. But I tried to back up Kirsten's position, by suggesting that she was under so much observation and scientifically-controlled medical intervention, that it was making her uncomfortable, to the point of inhibiting her ability to recover.

Dr Adams was very good. He said he would also make enquiries into alternative forms of treatment for her other than the ICU, such as a move back on to Hawthorn Ward. He was even willing to look into the possibility of her going home, with district nurses visiting to administer the medication. However, he did hold genuine reservations as to whether such nurses would be willing and able to take responsibility for such a serious case as Kirsten's, and he would personally not recommend this option.

On his leaving the room, I felt that the air had been cleared and that Kirsten was now in no doubt about the severity of her predicament. It turned out that this was the first time that anyone had made it clear to her exactly what she was doing in the ICU, and how difficult it was going to be for her to return to good health. As the seriousness of the situation hit us both, I felt like crying long and hard for all that we had experienced and all that the future might still hold in store.

I decided to go to our local health food shop and to try and see Dawn, a manager there who Kirsten had become friendly with, and ask her to give a holistic practitioner's view. I found Dawn and relayed all of Kirsten's sad, challenging tale. Dawn was visibly shocked and immediately became very caring. She advised me on protein drinks and handed me – without charge – a huge bottle of natural vitamin tablets. With this great battery of natural foods, I felt very much that this was a significant turning point in the course of Kirsten's road to health.

I got back to the ICU, and on giving Kirsten all of the good energy from Dawn, she was so moved that she burst into tears. The rest of the time was spent being with Kirsten while she ate almond butter and oatcakes, and sipped on juice fortified with the various protein powders that I had brought her over the previous few days. I stayed with Kirsten until the evening and felt happy that everything possible was being done for her.

The next morning, Sunday 16 August, I arrived at 9 a.m. The nurse on duty, Elena, refused to let me in, since it was before the start of visiting hours. This made me furious because Kirsten was relying on me to feed her, and I was being treated like an irritating interloper. Elena took my bag of food and allowed me in at 10 a.m. I was pleased to find that Kirsten was in good spirits and thinking positively about her situation, despite the fact that she'd had a strange chest pain in the middle of the night and had been given an ECG.

The time came for Dr Adams to visit Kirsten once more for the morning consultation. He told us that he had looked into the possibility of district nurses caring for Kirsten at home and it was a potential, if difficult option. He had also contacted Hawthorn Ward about admitting Kirsten who, having reflected on her own condition, acquiesced that this was the best option for now.

After he left, having formed a more viable working relationship with Elena, I helped tidy Kirsten's food cupboard, made sure she was comfortable, and headed on to perform in an afternoon choir concert. Little did I know that moving Kirsten to Hawthorn Ward had become much more than an idea, and that this would be the last time I would see Kirsten in her ICU environment.

PART 2

INTENSIVE CARE:
MY STORY

States of delirium

I am extremely fortunate that Trevor kept such a detailed diary account of my time in the ICU for me, the vast majority of which he recorded as events unfolded. Although I can remember a few bits and pieces from my first two days back in hospital, like talking to Sandra and the painful rides in the ambulance, otherwise my memories pretty much ended then completely. Despite the fact that I was clearly awake, speaking and even texting during the first two days, I can no longer recall any of the sequence of events. Nor do I have any recollection of the majority of Trevor's descriptions of my first week and a half in the ICU, even when I was supposedly communicating non-verbally with him and others. The first events depicted that I can remember with some degree of clarity occurred on 11 August, a full twelve days after my re-admittance to hospital.

I suppose it would be weird enough not having any memory of anything Trevor described, such as me waving my arms, squeezing hands and so on, and that instead, everything was just blank. I wish I could say it was so, like a blackout, or mornings when you awake and don't remember your dreams. But unfortunately, for most of the time I was in the ICU, I was convinced very different things were going on than actually were. And unlike dreams, which swiftly fade away over the course of the day, for me, one of the stranger elements about what follows is that whatever images or fantasies my mind conjured up are as clear to me now as they were then.

It was six months after leaving hospital that I was finally given an explanation for why this situation occurred: I was suffering an extreme form of delirium, which can cause fantasies, hallucinations, agitation and memory loss, among other things. It's apparently very common in patients in intensive care, particularly those who have been on a ventilator. In my case, the delirium was compounded by how severely ill I was with sepsis and the resultant medication and treatments. Its extremity meant that I was hallucinating right up until the end of my time in the ICU. Interestingly, once I was transferred to a regular ward, all of the delirium instantly stopped.

Swimming in the pod

It's difficult to say how long I was floating around in my fantasy world, or to allocate a time frame for what I believe happened and when. Some of my fantasies corresponded somewhat loosely with events in my actual circumstances, so I can now, with Trevor's help, pinpoint what some of them related to, but otherwise the time frame is pretty sketchy.

I'd like to say that I left my body and went off down a tunnel, into a blue light, or at least had some profound and life-affirming experiences. I'd like to say that, but instead, the fantasies I had bore some correlation to my existing life but not in any insightful, restful or meaningful ways.

I suppose the nearest I came to being in another dimension was at the beginning, probably corresponding to the first days I was unconscious, when I was effectively what I came to term 'swimming in a pod'. I don't know how to relate this experience, except that I seemed to be floating in water – presumably warm – but not feeling wet, and I was still able to breathe and talk at the same time. It was a feeling of weightlessness and being able to travel anywhere I wanted to essentially by rolling around, kind of somersaulting. Trevor was there with me much of the time and we were having conversations. It was an incredibly freeing situation, at least initially.

Wandering and sleep

Other times, when I wasn't in water, I was still seemingly floating around. At least, I seemed to drift around the hospital in a kind of weightless way. I think I was mostly aware that I was in hospital, but at times the hospital took on the appearance of a sort of cultural centre, which could even have been someone's house, and there were lots of people coming for social or educational events. One of the best night's sleep I perceived I had was curling up in a corner somewhere in this house.

That was another thing – the sense that I was being moved around a lot, and I developed this preoccupation of having to find somewhere to sleep every night. I'm sure this corresponded with many of my fitful sleeps, but the perception that either I was being moved or was in different places is one of the strongest themes. Trevor has repeatedly reassured me that, other than for tests or surgery, I never left the room or even the bed I was in, but I had the sensation of wandering around the hospital, effectively trying to find rest.

Oral history project

But back to swimming in the pod. At some point in my fantasy, I was made aware that my time in hospital was being resented – that I was, in effect, taking up space that someone else could occupy. The only way for me to stay was to justify my being there by coming up with an interesting project to do. I really fretted about this (and also for Trevor, whose presence was similarly in peril but, despite the fact he never did come up with a project, he seemed to have been allowed to stay). Eventually I hit upon the idea of reviving an oral history project I had worked on several years earlier, based in Cardiff. I thought it would be a good idea to re-interview some of the participants to see where they were now. I seemed to have been given the go-ahead and was very enthusiastic about it. I remember trying to gather recording equipment and to make contact with some of the people I intended to interview again, and basically was feeling energised with a new project under my belt.

While undertaking this endeavour, where I was located seemed to fluctuate. Other than a brief sojourn to a hot, rocky place, most of the time I seemed to be aware that I was in England, but even then, I thought there must have been a few hot, sunny days that August. However, Trevor has assured me that the way my room was positioned, I would not have been aware of any sun coming through and, in any case, the ICU was kept at a cool temperature. There was one afternoon when I remember Trev (truthfully) giving me ice water dipped in a flannel and putting it on my head. I thought it was because we were going through a heatwave, but it turns out it's likely that I was the heatwave – i.e. having a fever. I don't remember actually going out to do the interviewing itself but at least my position in the hospital was secure.

There's a strange postscript to this particular fantasy. I've had sporadic contact with my supervisor from this project since it ended a few years ago, but nothing directly relating to the project itself for some time now. The last time I'd emailed him had been about five months earlier. But somehow, without him knowing anything that had happened to me, he emailed me in the middle of August to say that he was archiving this project and asked me if I had copies of a couple of the interviews which he was missing. Very strange indeed.

Actor Joseph

I had another aspect of a fantasy later 'coming true' in real life. This incident involved a nurse called Joseph, who I thought was an actor. In fact, I was convinced they were shooting a film at the hospital, some kind of *Star Wars*-like epic. I became very annoyed because I felt I was being confined to my bed so as not to disrupt the film set, and that everyone was becoming very obsessed with the film and not getting on with their proper jobs at the hospital.

One of the main actors was a wiry, black man called Joseph, and we had a very in-depth conversation about various things, including where he was from in Africa, and what it was like living in London and how cold it gets in Canada – all very plausible, credible topics. However, I remember he kept looking at his phone, which I thought was him checking when he needed to be on the set. I was pleased at what a nice and down-to-earth person he was for such an established actor.

Months later, at home, I remember seeing the trailer for the new *Star Wars* film and was amazed when one of the main actors – unlike any in the previous series – turned out to be John Boyega, a London-based actor born of Nigerian parents. I don't expect he ever spent much time working in a hospital, though…

Stuart and Super Dan

Most of my fantasies had some correlation with reality and involved people in the hospital, if not exactly in the roles in which they were employed. For example, I acutely remember the nurses Stuart, and one I insisted on calling 'Super Dan', presumably because of his considerably large build. During the second week when I was speaking again, I remember always being pleased when they were on duty, and exclaiming every time I'd see them: 'It's Stuart! It's Super Dan!' and them always being very friendly and kind to me.

This seems especially odd since one of my fantasies involved being a bit of a party animal (and trust me, this is *pure* fantasy) and, as the story went, I would get drunk and be scantily clad. It was Stuart and Super Dan's job to bundle me into the back of some kind of lorry and effectively tie me down, so I wouldn't escape. Being in party mode, I was always very happy to see them and greeted them loudly, and I didn't seem to mind being manhandled and tied down, either because I was bladdered or because I knew they were my friends and rescuers. I'm not sure how many times I had this fantasy but I know now that they must have corresponded to the times I was physically restrained, especially the night I was tied to the bed to stop me pulling out my arterial lines.

Getting out of bed

Because Stuart and Super Dan were around a lot, they probably morphed more and more into their real roles, and more of the contact with them related to what was actually occurring. One thing I do remember is asking Stuart to help me get out of the bed. As soon as I was extubated, this became a bit of an obsession of mine, and as soon as I could speak, I was constantly asking people to help me to get out of bed. Of course, they all refused – even Stuart, however kindly. I think my intense desire to get out of the bed was a combination of being in pain (even a nurse later commented how uncomfortable these beds were) and feeling intensely restless.

Sleep was not something I ever did much of in the ICU, as I was always awake for one reason or another – being too hot or cold or uncomfortable. There was one night I insisted on being allowed to sit in the chair in the room and, of course, I needed help even to get up, let alone out of the bed and over to a chair. My constant pleas that night were regularly refused by a male and female nursing double-act, who repeated in turn: 'It's not safe, it's not safe – you have to sleep.' This was then followed by my repeated demands for my computer. I find it crazy now that I was so sick and could barely move, yet my mind was super alert and needed stimulation and contact with the outside world. (Ironically, when I was finally given my computer in the early hours of the morning – in bed – it was only to discover there was no functioning Wi-Fi network and not much I could do on it other than write messages in Word.)

Painkillers at night

Most of the nurses were incredibly kind, patient and very helpful. Some of them I remember quite well, along with their caring natures, but I've been further amazed through reading Trevor's diary at the sheer extent of this care. I think most of my difficult issues happened at night, and occasionally with less happy results. The worst night I can remember in the ICU was when I was (for some reason) in so much pain that I kept calling out for a nurse, begging repeatedly for someone to 'please help me, please…' The nurse on duty that night was unfortunately one of the few that was not very nice, and she eventually shouted at me to shut up, that she had too many people to look after to keep attending to me.

This nurse was truly the exception and, not to detract from the assiduous care that the nurses dispensed, but I do have to say that once I became aware of it, the frequency with which painkillers were offered – especially at night – was incredible. As soon as I called for a nurse, I would first of all be offered painkillers – a whole array of them, depending on your preference. One of the painkillers regularly dispensed was called Oramorph – a kind of liquid morphine, which I took very often. Sometimes I took the painkillers even when I wasn't in pain but was desperate to sleep, and hoped one of them would help knock me out.

Most of the time they didn't work, and I only ever remember getting a few hours' sleep a night. The blankets were very thin and did not keep you warm so I often slept in a sweater. But, because I was so ill, I would get feverish, so I was either too hot or too cold. One time towards the end I remember accepting paracetamol and waking up in a terrible sweat and having to remove half my clothing, having finally been allowed to replace the hospital gown with my own comfortable jogging gear.

Muslim family

Despite what must have been a hive of constant activity on the ward, I was strangely unaware of other patients, pretty much until the weekend I left intensive care, with one notable exception. My field of vision would have been limited to the two rooms across the hall from me. In one of them, I distinctly remember seeing a dark-skinned family that could have been from many parts of the world, but that I, at least, convinced myself were Muslim. Trevor confirmed that there was indeed such a family, Muslim or otherwise, at least for a short time, if not for the longer period I thought they were there. I became convinced that there was a young boy who was a patient, and was quite moved that the room had been 'specially decorated' for him, with mobiles above the bed. (These, I later learned, were actually mounted brackets and were exactly the same in every room.) I thought there was a particular room on the ward where the men went to pray, as I saw them disappear through a door (which was probably the exit).

Once, I had a dark-skinned male nurse with grey hair and a trimmed beard who, in addition to keeping an eye on me (since I was awake most of the night), I decided had the responsibility for providing Halal food for this Muslim family, which came sealed and wrapped, and which he dispensed through this special bright yellow unit. On later inspection, I discovered that what I thought was a food-dispensing unit was in fact the hazardous waste bin. I similarly became preoccupied with these massive orange sheets on a roller in the room, which I thought were comprised of pressed pumpkin. These turned out to be orange disposable plastic aprons the nurses tore off of a roll and disposed of after a single use – hence the need for there to be so much pumpkin in the room!

Room decorating

As mentioned, I was in a constant state of delirium for pretty much the whole time I was in the ICU. My regular hallucinations continued right up until my very last night in intensive care, when I was once again wandering around looking for somewhere to sleep. This time I was in what seemed like a cinema or a church, with rows and rows of seating. I agreed to stretch out across some seats and sleep there. This was made difficult because there was a lot of activity going on, what seemed to be teams of people bringing in building and decorating supplies and working on a room some distance across from me. I realised they must have been redecorating the children's room (where the Muslim boy had been). I do remember thinking it was strange it was happening at night, but thought perhaps this was the best time for it, even though it was clearly raining outside, which must have made it difficult bringing things in from the ambulance parked outside.

In the morning, I became less convinced about the redecorating, and asked the sweet nurse Amy about it, as it didn't seem as likely to me as it did in the night. She very kindly confirmed that they weren't decorating a room but instead bringing in lots of medical equipment during the night (though not from outside in the rain) for a patient who needed it. It was the first time I'd overtly questioned one of the medical staff about what I thought was occurring around me, and genuinely realised that things weren't entirely as I thought they were.

Listening in

Strangely, even when I was seeing plenty of things that weren't there, my auditory function and general awareness of my own physical circumstances seemed to return much more readily. The first day I can be absolutely sure of an incident, and one which tallies with Trevor's account, is on 11 August. Trevor talked about a lovely Irish nurse, Claire, and how good she was with me. Though visually the room seemed like a different place to me (more like a classroom), I remember something about her interacting with me while I chewed on the intubation tube.

But most of all, what I remember (in much greater detail than Trevor does), is the conversation the two of them had about her family's farm in Ireland, where she was headed that weekend. I was deeply touched by her heartfelt description of her bucolic home setting. As the blessed Einaudi music went round and round in a loop, I also distinctly remember thinking, I hope you get there soon, if only to get away from this incessantly repetitive music. So, clearly my personality and even sense of humour returned pretty quickly, despite my uncertainty about what I was perceiving around me.

Extubation

Though I don't recall the actual extubation process, I clearly remember the physiotherapist coming to see me with Scott, the anaesthetist. Trevor would not have been present for this and so did not record her pummelling me very hard in various places to determine if I was physically ready to get out of bed, something I had been desperate to do forever. So, although I was a bit surprised by all of this thrashing, I submitted to whatever she said and did. I was pulled and pressed on so hard I was thinking that I would not want to meet this woman in a dark alley at night. But then I remember the immense weightlessness and relief of being freed of the intubation tube, though, of course, I was still hooked up to various monitoring machines. I know I found it fairly difficult to speak for several days, as my voice was quite hoarse and fluctuated regularly.

Following the extubation, my nutritional intake began to be monitored and acutely assessed. The main clinical obsession was for me to get my protein levels up as quickly as possible. Though the medical team would have preferred feeding me through an NJ tube and had encountered little experience of veganism, incredibly, they acquiesced to letting Trevor buy whatever food I needed. I think they were pleasantly surprised by how aware we were of products out there on the market, but I had been a healthy vegan for over twenty years by that stage. I know I certainly didn't feel like eating much but felt like I had to make an effort, if only to keep the medical team and NJ tube off of me. I even ordered a meal from the hospital – once –

the ill-fated Asian meal, which my body told me immediately it was not prepared to digest. But I do remember with some small pleasure sitting on my high-backed 'throne' eating what I could by way of protein shakes, soya yogurt, almond butter and oatcakes. I also remember the comic episode of the blueberries rolling around on the otherwise spotless floor.

Gary

Speaking of spotless, there was a cleaner I remember very well, once I was awake and interacting with people. This delicate-looking young man, Gary, was often on duty, meticulously cleaning my room and all of the medical equipment. (It was a strange experience having someone clean around you, while you lie immobile in a bed.) He was always very pleasant, though he seemed quite dour and kept to himself. I always said hello and thanked him when he left, but that was about the extent of our interaction, until one day I charged Trevor with the task of seeing if he could make the young lad smile. So, Trevor engaged him in a conversation and found out about him and his young son, whom he doted on. Once he got talking to us he was quite friendly and sweet. He was very moved by our situation, and especially by Trevor's dedication in coming to sit with me every day, all day. 'Yours is a true love story,' he said one time. I suppose in a way, it was.

The chemical pod

I would say that Friday 14 August was the first day I could truly remember being present the whole day. From the morning, I had two lovely nurses looking after me, a sturdy Polish nurse called Paulina, and a pretty Caribbean nurse called Grace. I remember them giving me a bed wash (considering I couldn't wash properly, the nurses kept me meticulously clean during my stay there). I started to cry because I thought I was going to be in hospital forever and that I was never going to be allowed to leave. At that stage, I still didn't know or understand what was wrong with me. I just knew that I had an infection and wasn't able to leave hospital. Paulina reassured me and urged me to focus on getting better. She was extremely caring and kind.

Paulina and I had a long (and lucid) conversation about her life in Poland, and I even offered her my few words in Polish and told her about my experiences living there over ten years earlier. Grace and I talked about Caribbean food, and she blissfully freed me from my oxygen mask and gave me a nasal cannula I could put in my nostrils instead, which was much less hot and cumbersome. I think this was the first day I was fully aware of all the wires sticking out from all over me and that I was attached to a machine, so that if I wanted to go to the loo, the machine had to come with me.

Paulina, Grace and I spent all day in what I termed 'the chemical pod'. Although this space seemed quite different to Claire's 'classroom' and the 'film set', this appellation isn't as illogical as it might at first seem. At some point a notice went up on the door saying, 'STOP Isolationist Zone', and advising people to wash, as they were now entering an infected area. The doors were closed much of the day, which reinforced the sense of being cut off from the rest of the ward.

Around midday, while Trevor was off food shopping, Mr Ellis came round and wanted to discuss the possibility of surgery, or what he termed 'a full pelvic clearance' as the best option of ridding my body of infection. I was very upset and panicked and told him I would not discuss anything with him until Trevor was present too. He agreed to return with Sandra after lunch. I felt quite threatened, and even a little afraid of Mr Ellis. I called Trevor and told him Ellis was on the rampage and urged him to come back as soon as possible.

Trevor returned, followed by Ellis and Sandra, who seemed to descend from a spiral staircase. Trevor has subsequently explained to me that a fixing bracket coming down from the ceiling behind me could have resembled a spiralling staircase, and that the two doctors went to the computer behind me first and came round to the bed, which could have created the illusion of them coming down the stairs.

Even in my groggy state, I was adamantly against any more surgery. Fortunately, Trevor presented a much more articulate case against it, along the lines of his preference for me coming out of this whole situation as physically close as possible to the way I went in. Thankfully, they seemed willing to consider this. What I remember most is plucking up the courage to say in a very heartfelt, if strangled way, to Ellis, who had performed the initial surgery, 'At very least, you owe me an apology.'

The bid to escape

As mentioned, I still had no real idea what had happened to me or what I was doing in the ICU. All I knew was that I had some kind of infection, which had resulted from the original surgery in some way, and which necessitated me staying in hospital under intense monitoring and given regular medication. I think it was the persistent monitoring of everything that went in and out of me, along with the pressure to get my nutrition levels up, that really stressed me out. I felt that if I didn't get out soon, I never would.

By the Saturday morning, I was desperate to go home. When Trevor arrived in the morning, I begged him to plead my case to the doctor to allow me to go home, arguing that I wasn't going to get any better under this constant scrutiny in the ICU, in a sterile, soulless environment with machines constantly beeping. He said he would do his best to support me. I spent the morning being anxious about where the doctor was and keen not to miss him on his rounds.

That morning we had a new doctor in charge called Dr Adams. Without any preamble, I immediately put my case to him: that in order for me to get better I was going to need to do so at home; that I didn't feel sick enough to be in intensive care, but if I stayed any longer I certainly would be. It was to his credit that he listened to me and didn't rule out my wishes before putting forward his own suggestions. He very calmly explained to me that I had the kind of infection that needed constant monitoring and IV antibiotics, which could be difficult – though not impossible – to administer from home. He said there were district nurses who could possibly fill this role, but he would have to look into the logistics of this. He was also concerned that I could end up back in hospital again in a much worse state than before. As such, he very plainly advised against the notion of me going home at that stage.

Instead, he put forward a sort of halfway house option of me transferring to a regular ward, which might help me to feel a bit more normal. He agreed that there wasn't anything specific that the ICU was doing that couldn't be done on a regular ward. He warned me that there wouldn't be the one-to-one nursing care available, and I would likely have to wait longer if I needed something. But on the plus side, there would be an opportunity for me to have a shower, and I might feel more comfortable in a more 'normal' hospital environment.

He had me at the word 'shower'. After two weeks, I was desperate to have a proper wash and to shampoo my incredibly tangled hair. I agreed to this option straight away, even though the regular ward in question would be the gynaecological Hawthorn Ward, where I had started out, and I would transfer to being under the direct care of Mr Ellis. I was a bit daunted by this, as he was effectively, as I saw it, the man who had put me in the ICU in the first place, and was now pushing for a surgical 'full pelvic clearance'. But I was so desperate to escape that I accepted that being under his clutches again was the condition of getting out of the ICU, and thought that I would find a way to deal with this when the time came.

I also felt a strange deadline to flee the ICU before the more relaxed weekend atmosphere in the hospital gave way to the return of the intense forensic monitoring on Monday, with the dietician weighing up protein measurements and the ever-present threat of an NJ tube being fitted. I was done with tubes and constant monitoring and acceded that a regular ward would be the best place for me.

After Dr Adams left, I felt a small sense of hope that I would finally be free of this nightmare scenario. It was then that I asked Trevor to clarify exactly what my situation was. Until that point, Trevor didn't realise that I had retained no memories after my first day and a half back in hospital, even though I was still conscious and communicating until the time I went back into surgery. I had no idea what I was doing in intensive care, nor why any of the medical team hadn't explained anything to me. The odd doctor may have done so to some degree and I may not have taken anything in, but it was Trevor's thorough explanation that followed which was the first time I absorbed any detailed information regarding my condition. It was the first time I'd heard, for example, that I'd been in a coma for nearly two weeks. I found this very difficult to accept.

I then began questioning Trevor about my various fantasy situations, asking him to confirm whether any of these things had actually happened. I was amazed when he replied 'no' to each and every one of them. I just couldn't believe that none of the world I had created in my head had ever existed. It took me a long time to process this and to find my way through the fog.

Shortly after this frank discussion, Trevor shared with me all of the 'Get Well' cards and email messages from my friends. I was grateful that he had been keeping in touch with everyone on my behalf. I started to realise that there were people I had arranged to meet and places I had organised to go, and that somehow this time had passed and I had never contacted any of these people to offer an explanation for my absence. It was extremely fortunate that Trevor had stepped in and filled them in on what had happened, albeit in somewhat vague terms. Then out came his big, grey gym bag – full of cuddly toys! Trevor had brought a bunch of them from home, including the poor, neglected Chubb Chubb, with whom I had a joyful reunion.

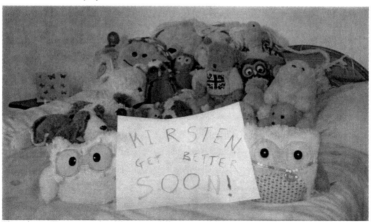

The photo Trevor took with my cuddly toys, which I eventually saw that Saturday. The infamous Chubb Chubb is on the left.

I can also say that this was the first day I truly became aware of my surroundings, seeing the room as it actually was, including the 'story board' with details about me propped up in the corner. I remember watching visitors pass through the hallway, and can also very safely say that the sun was shining through the windows that day, as I recall the woman in the room across from me sitting in beams of sunlight, reading the paper and looking oddly content.

Mobility

That Saturday was also the first day I gained any degree of mobility. I have Amy the nurse to thank for that. By this stage, my muscles had become so weak that I couldn't stand or move without help. Earlier in the day I remember having to wait almost half an hour to go to the loo because I needed a nurse to help me get there, and she was busy elsewhere on the ward. When Amy came on shift later in the day, she brought me a walker and showed me how to get up from the bed, positioning myself in front of it and leaning on it for balance. I could only walk as far as the chair in the room or to the loo and back before I had to sit down again, but it was a start. It felt like an incredible gain for me, literally my first step towards any kind of independence.

That night, I awoke in the middle of the night with a pain in my chest. I didn't think that much of it, but pushed the call button just to ask Amy about it. The next thing I knew a doctor appeared with an ECG machine and put electrodes around my chest and took measurements. The doctor sat at the desk in the room – with the lamp on – for quite a while making notes, and then the whole process was repeated a couple of hours later. I remember wondering what all the fuss was about over a small chest pain. I suppose if I had truly understood anything about the severity of my condition, I would have realised why they weren't taking any chances.

Leaving the ICU

Sunday morning saw me put under the care of an overbearing, bossy nurse called Elena, who was similarly short with the other nurses and constantly insisted on doing things her way. She refused to let me get out of bed myself, despite my having learned to use the walker to get around myself the day before. She kept repeating that it wasn't safe and that I must ask for help if I wanted to get up. I remember lying there very upset, seething about this small bit of freedom being taken away from me.

However, it was Elena's briskness that I have to thank for my getting out of the ICU that day. She brought her considerable experience to the fore and ended up being a powerhouse of efficiency, because once my transfer to Hawthorn Ward was authorised, the wheels turned very swiftly, and this Amazonian-like nurse was instrumental in it coming to pass. There was something like three hours between the transfer being confirmed and when the transport was to collect me, and there was a mountain of paperwork to deal with in between, as well as all of my intravenous lines having to be removed, which thankfully Elena was able to do.

Then, all of my things had to be packed up to be taken away. Unusually, Trevor was away during all of these preparations because he had a concert that he had committed to performing in. It's a real shame he wasn't there, because it ended up being Elena and another man who 'packed' all of my things which, by now, were all over the room in a disorderly fashion. Everything had to be done quickly because time was ticking on before the transport would arrive. Since Elena refused to let me get out of bed, I had to sit and watch helplessly as all my personal things were shoved into bags willy-nilly. The worst of this was when this other man opened up the gym bag containing all of the cuddly toys and, after expressing amused surprise at them, proceeded to pack my food *on top of them*, including – and this makes me shudder to this day – an *opened* carton of grape juice, which was in a flimsy plastic bag. Incredibly, none of the animals got saturated, as the juice mostly sloshed into the plastic bag.

Mercifully, I had the very white Chubb Chubb with me in the bed, who Elena unceremoniously tossed onto my chest, saying 'Don't forget this!' The impact winded me a bit as Chubby weighs a ton, which immediately put me in mind of my chest pains the night before. I was musing that it would have been kind of funny (and rather embarrassing) if, while the team were in and out with the ECG machine, it turned out I had just been lying the wrong way on the very heavy Chubbster.

Since I wasn't able to get out of bed, I also never got a chance to explore the ward, to at least see what it looked like from outside the room, something I was planning to try and do that day with my walker. I desperately wanted to see how I could have conjured up all of those fantasies of rooms, compared to what was actually there in reality. When the transport came, I asked if I could have a quick look around in the wheelchair.

Even though we were still waiting for a doctor to come and sign my discharge papers, as the transport team were on a tight schedule, they were reluctant to leave the confines of the room. So I left the ICU without any clearer understanding of what it really looked like, something I think would have helped me to process my experience there. (Seven months later, I was invited back to the ICU and managed to see my exact room, since it was unoccupied, and it was surprisingly pretty much how I had remembered it.)

However, at the time, I was bustled out of the ICU by a very harassed transport team. What I do remember is being wheeled through a series of long and winding corridors. It all passed by very quickly, and I couldn't get a sense of the vast space, but I remember thinking what a trek it must have been for Trevor to get here, though he's since told me that he would have come via a different route.

The second surprise was when we were in the lift, which had mirrors (whose idea was that – putting mirrors in hospital lifts?) I couldn't believe the face looking back at me, which I hadn't seen since I had entered hospital. I was ghost white with big, dark brown hollowed-out eyes and my hair, now tangled and frizzy, was pulled back from my face, which accentuated my pallor. Yes, a truly gothic look, though, once I got over the shock, I kidded people that I was too early for Halloween. In the coming weeks, when the medical team commented on how much better I looked, I shuddered to think how truly deathly I must have looked before.

PART 3
LIFE ON THE WARD

FIRST DAYS

I was taken to Hawthorn Ward, where I had come for my original day surgery, and which was a unit designated for gynaecological procedures. It was an older building consisting of one long corridor, with rooms off to either side, and an operating theatre at the end. At the entrance is the reception and nursing station, and I immediately recalled my initial return to hospital, when I had sat in agony for an hour, waiting for someone to see me.

This time I was brought straight in, and was pleasantly surprised to be given my own room, though I wasn't sure why. I thought maybe my story had done the rounds, and they wanted to give me some peace and quiet. It's far more likely that since I had such a serious infection they were keeping me in isolation for my own protection, as well as for the other patients. I later thought it was because I was due to be there for an indefinite period, rather than most of the women who were in and out in a matter of days. As it turned out, I was in the ward for two and a half weeks overall.

Whatever the reason, I was incredibly grateful to be in a room on my own. It was a lovely room with big trees outside, and for the first time in weeks I could see birds. I was so relieved to be there – away from the intensity of the ICU. The nurses were very welcoming, although the only thing I requested was a walker, and one particular nurse was surprisingly dismissive, and said with it being a weekend they didn't know where they would get one. This got me very upset and depressed, because I had just learned to walk again the day before and was otherwise too unsteady to walk without a walker. So I effectively had to sit on the bed once again, immobile. Fortunately, an hour or so later a walker did appear and I was very grateful, as it meant I could go to the loo on my own or walk around the ward, though as I was very weak and tired, I didn't attempt to leave my room until the next day.

Trevor has a record of me sending him the following text upon arrival: 'Hi T. Entered another parallel universe via bed 12 tho this time am v awake + looking at trees. Hope aft has gone well. Looking forward to settling in.'

Trevor arrived later that afternoon, following his concert, which had gone very well, and sat with me until later that evening. The rest of the day and into the night I had a steady stream of medical visitors to my room, which ended at about 2 a.m. I honestly didn't know what all of the fuss was about. I was used to being hot and cold and generally feeling unwell. I didn't feel any different than I had before and didn't know why I merited all of this attention, especially when I'd been told to expect a lot less personal care on a regular ward compared to the ICU. The visits included regular monitoring of my vital signs, such as my heart rate and blood pressure, and it seemed as though everything had gone up.

Everyone was especially perturbed by my high temperature – generally measuring in at 38.7 – and all had very authoritative words to say about my case, though, with it being weekend staff, most of them I never saw again. Many of them were incredibly young and looked fresh out of medical school. One of these young doctors seemed unhappy about me being there and was keen to send me back to the ICU. Thankfully, it seemed that they eventually got clearance from someone in authority in the ICU that, as I wasn't likely to die on their watch, it was okay for me to stay.

Trevor and I later talked about this first day back in the ward, and since acquiring my medical notes, I now know how 'medically ill' I was deemed to be, and how unprepared the ward was to deal with me in the state I was in. It's a miracle that they agreed to admit me and let me stay.

In between all of these visits on the first day, I attempted to call my mum in Canada. Now that I was back in the 'real world', I became aware that I hadn't spoken to her for several weeks. Today was Sunday, when she sometimes went to visit my brother and his kids in the suburbs, but I thought, in light of my own situation, that she might have been home. Trev called on his mobile but the phone rang and rang. We tried a bit later and it was the same again. I started to get worried about her, which was ironic, given my own situation. Trevor emailed my brother, who wrote back straight away and explained that they had been having a belated third birthday party for their son, my nephew. I felt sad to be missing all of the festivities. He said that our mum was likely to be home in an hour.

When I finally reached her, the conversation was quite surreal. She talked non-stop about the party and what the cake was like and who ate what food. She seemed oddly unaware of my predicament, which I eventually tried to make her tune into. She took it in somewhat, but not entirely, as remains the case to this day. Anyway, I was glad to be able to talk to her (well, mostly listen), and reassure her that I was out of serious danger.

One of the doctors – another one who I never saw again – decided to put me on a saline drip all night to try and hydrate me. All I can say is it was like having an icy claw holding on to my hand all night – a most horrible sensation. She wanted to repeat it early that morning but fortunately, when she appeared, I happened to be on the phone with Trevor. He spoke to her and managed to convince her not to repeat it, on the grounds that my chest was at that time very vulnerable to infection, and introducing further liquids could have increased the risk of a chest infection. I'm glad that she subsequently cancelled the drip as I most certainly would not have agreed to it again.

That morning when I woke up, I looked out the window to the trees and the birds and it was then, in my weakened, debilitated state, that I decided I was going to get better. I remember looking out at the quite pastoral scene and thinking about the birds at home that I had been feeding, and all of the animals that needed help in the world, which has always been my passion. With this came the feeling that I needed to get out of hospital and get on with things, to pursue my mission and carry on with my life. I felt this very clearly, very confidently, in spite of what everyone else seemed to be thinking to the contrary about my current state. I just knew I had to ignite my own healing and recovery from within.

With this in mind, I resolutely approached an attempt at showering. The afternoon before, after I had settled in, I attempted to wash my hair, which was in a particularly terrible state. I don't think it had been washed properly in two weeks and it was completely tangled, like a bird's nest. I remember one nurse in the ICU trying to comb it – bless her – but it was a pretty impossible task. However, I was too weak to stand up so I remember I sat at the sink and tried to wash it, and put every 'Curly Girl' product into it that I could muster. It would take a couple of weeks for it to start resembling anything like it did before, but it was a good start.

The next day, my first morning in the ward, I was buoyed by the fact that there was a shower where you could sit down, as I was still too weak to stand still for more than a few seconds unaided. I managed to get myself to the shower with my walker but found it too hard to use, and after drenching myself and all of my stuff, I had to get some nurses to help me. It made me realise, once again, how weak and dependent I was, and I was immensely grateful for their kindness. Even afterwards, I was still covered from my neck to my abdomen in bits of medical adhesive tape which had held down a variety of tubes and equipment, and which made me look like a Polynesian warrior festooned with tattoos. I discovered that it would take a long time to get rid of it all.

Later that morning, after I was back in a fresh hospital gown, I was reflecting that, while Trevor was continuing to feed me – that morning he had very kindly brought me a morning smoothie and a tub of fruit, I thought perhaps I should try and relieve the burden on him bringing me all of my food and see if there was anything on the hospital menu that I could eat. With this in mind, armed with my walker, I went in search of Pat, one of the health care workers I'd become friendly with, and pootled slowly up the corridor, as I saw her standing at the nurses' station.

I was so focused on getting to her and asking about ordering a salad for lunch that I didn't even notice Mr Ellis standing behind the desk, until he exclaimed in complete shock, 'Is that Kirsten Lavine I see before me?' to which I replied dully, 'Some version, yes.' I was still disgusted with my general state and condition, whereas he was flabbergasted that I was already up and walking around. The last time he'd seen me was a few days before in the ICU 'chemical pod'. He'd heard that I'd been transferred to Hawthorn Ward, but this was the first time he'd seen me.

Ellis later came into my room and sat on a chair by the edge of the bed. He said, very humbly, that he'd been thinking about what I'd said all weekend, that I deserved an apology, and that he'd really taken this to heart. He said, 'I'm sorry this has happened to you. We're not in the habit of putting patients into intensive care.' At the time, Trev and I thought they were directly responsible for what went wrong, and though I appreciated the apology, I didn't think it went quite far enough. But given his esteemed position in the hospital, it must have taken a lot for him to offer even that.

He then laid out the various options regarding treatment. The first was to continue administering antibiotics in a sort of war of attrition, hoping it would be enough to wear down the infection eventually. Then there was some talk of a drainage procedure, though I wasn't exactly sure what this entailed. Ellis said that the option of a full pelvic clearance was looking less necessary than before, but it remained in the background as an option. I was so weary that I really wanted as little interference as possible. I also remember talking about when I would be back on my bicycle again, and Ellis assured me it would be within six months. As it turned out, it was within six weeks!

That morning, it was discovered that I had also developed a deep vein thrombosis (DVT), or what's commonly known as a blood clot, in my left leg. I had complained about pain in this leg towards the end of my stay in the ICU, and I suppose as a result, I was taken over to the main building for testing. I remember sitting in the waiting room with mostly elderly people, and lamenting to this very nice, no-nonsense nurse called Kathy, that I was never going to get better, and her assuring me very sincerely that I would.

As my wheelchair had gone back with the ambulance crew, they had to source another wheelchair to get me from the waiting room to the examining room, as I couldn't walk that far without a walker. I remember all the elderly people looking at me, perhaps wondering how I had got there. I felt pretty pitiful myself. The examination consisted of waving a wand very painfully up and down my legs, and they found a couple of minor clots in my lower left calf. From then on, I had to wear awkward embolic stockings which cut into my legs, and worse, I was stabbed every night with Clexane injections in the stomach for the next two weeks.

I had been on various different medications since being re-admitted to hospital, especially antibiotics, and I was currently on a powerful one called meropenem, which I had intravenously administered three times a day. I gathered that I had also acquired candida along the way, so I had to take something called fluconazole for it, which consisted of an IV bag which dripped through a tube into a cannula in my hand. I remember watching this thing drip, drip, drip at night, and because I was hooked up to a machine, I couldn't go to sleep until it stopped because I couldn't move without jerking it with me.

One of the worst things about being in hospital is feeling powerless regarding what medication you're told to take. Much of this medication was kept locked in a locker in my room. Medication names and doses seemed to change frequently and few explanations were ever offered, and certainly the side effects were never discussed.

I still don't know whether the hot and sweaty flushes and headaches I endured were from the infection or from all of the antibiotics I was given. I definitely never felt good after I'd taken them. I'm also assuming it was the antibiotics that made everything taste funny, and why I had such difficulty eating. It was quite stressful having my food intake monitored and being repeatedly told I had to eat more, whilst not being able to eat because of the medication.

However, there were certain treatments which I could refuse. For example, there was a horrible energy drink listed on my chart which, apart from its questionable contents, was not even vegan, and which was offered to me most days. Despite regularly refusing it, this continued, until I finally said that it shouldn't even be on my chart in the first place, only to be told that it couldn't be taken off until the doctors took it off, which thankfully one of them eventually did. Also, one night after taking paracetamol and waking up sweating like crazy, I had paracetamol crossed off permanently from my chart.

Ironically, while I seemed to be able to have access to painkillers whenever I wanted, it was as long as they came from a nurse who recorded my intake. I'll never forget the time that I confessed offhandedly to a nurse, who Trev and I subsequently nicknamed 'Bond girl', that I had just taken some ibuprofen which I'd had on me from home. She got very irate and demanded that I hand over my contraband drugs, which were then locked in my locker and never seen again, and not even given back to me when I left.

Later on, I asked Trevor (perhaps wrongly) to 'smuggle in' some ibuprofen so I could take it when I wanted and not have to wait for a nurse to be available to give me some. I kept this secret stash of ibuprofen hidden and never let on to the nurses that I had it. I hope the hospital police don't come after me now, and in any case, this 'illicit drug taking' doesn't seem to have impaired my recovery.

But joking aside, the medical team, especially the nurses, were right to monitor and record everything that was given to me. This meant that I ended up with a heavy, bulging file – over 500 pages when Trev and I later got hold of a copy of it, as the amount of paperwork involved in hospital procedures is enormous. Absolutely everything is recorded, from the time your temperature is taken, to the time of every pill you ever ingest. I also had something called a 'drug chart' which, for reasons unclear to me, was sometimes kept just *outside* my room. But many a day it would just float around, and a nurse would arrive ready to administer medication and then have to go and find my drug chart. Invariably someone would have borrowed it and was using it, or just hadn't put it back. I don't know where this chart went on its regular travels. Personally, I think it was so high on all the drugs it was on, it just floated around at whim.

PASSING THE DAYS

It was the regular monitoring and administration of drugs that contributed to a constant stream of people going in and out of my room all day. I don't know if this was the case with the other patients, although there were nurses who seemed to make regular rounds. For me, apart from the various medications I needed three times a day spaced apart at regular intervals, it seemed that most days, especially in the beginning, there was a steady flow of people in and out for one reason or another.

The way the room was set up, I could hear people knocking, but couldn't see who it was until a couple of seconds after they entered the room and walked towards the bed. It could be anyone from nurses doing regular observations and offering painkillers, to junior doctors expressing interest in my case, to the consultants on their rounds, to the nutritionist and pharmacist, or cleaners and health care workers, changing bedding and offering meals and water.

One thing I will say is that they took cleanliness and sterility very, very seriously. While I lay weakly in bed, the room and bathroom were cleaned thoroughly every day and were spotless. All the nurses and doctors were equally vigilant, and the majority washed their hands upon entering and leaving the room. A few days after I was admitted, an infection sign went up on my door, whereupon everyone entering would put on a new pair of latex rubber gloves and a plastic apron, both of which would be discarded after each visit.

Since there wasn't really any regular schedule, and I never knew who was coming and when, sometimes in the morning I wouldn't want to wash for fear of missing someone. I would often just wait until everyone I thought was coming had been before embarking on something like taking a shower and dressing. Of course, if I was in the bathroom they could have just come back, but since some of them were on such a tight schedule, if it was someone I needed to see or something I needed to hear then I would just sit tight and wait in bed.

But it was strange to have a steady stream of people, many of whom I had never seen before (and sometimes would not see again), and although I kept my door shut (hence the perfunctory knocking), everyone was allowed in at all times. I also got used to complete strangers asking me to expose my stomach with its web of angry scars and sores. I felt like some weird circus exhibit lying like a slab, as all manner of medical staff poked and prodded my abdomen, making noises and recording notes on a chart. I'm not sure if the enlarged cast of medical characters was partly to do with the fact that the two main consultants in charge of my care were intermittently on holiday, so other deputies came instead, but there did seem to be a wide range of different doctors visiting me from day to day.

How the doctors introduced themselves was also quite surprising. I was used to calling the nurses by their first names, but it felt strange that many of the doctors, particularly the younger ones, introduced themselves with their first names only. Even Sandra I always called by her first name. I found this familiarity very odd, and yet there was a peculiar sense of intimacy created by the intense care that I was still in need of. But it was something I found very strange and a bit hard to get used to.

Most of the doctors had an excellent bedside manner and listened seriously to what I had to say, no matter how inarticulately it may have come out. All of them were similarly very respectful of one another, and I never experienced any sense of anyone pulling rank or acting over-authoritatively. I found one doctor particularly admirable because when she said she was going to do something, she did it, and kept me duly informed. One time she wanted to have my observations done and said that rather than find a nurse, it would just be quicker if she did it herself. I was very impressed with this individual.

These 'obs', or observations, were done at regular four-hour intervals (two hours in the ICU), to check my blood pressure, respiration rate, heart rate and temperature. The nurses seemed to get very agitated if any of these were out of sorts and made prompt notes on a chart. I never felt like I was being told very much. I don't know if it was because the nurses weren't authorised to tell me, and instead were there primarily to carry out duties like taking blood and recording observations. I always dreaded these obs, as I always felt like I was in line to fail the next test.

Sometimes I would be given contradictory information on matters like when to wear the embolic stockings, or what medications were going to be administered or changed. It took me a while to sort out who was in charge and made the decisions – essentially the consultants – and then I usually reserved my questions or concerns for them. But it was very exhausting to be told different things a lot of the time.

It was also the consultants, who were around the least, who gave me any sense of the overall picture of my recovery, though even they tended to talk mainly in measurable medical terms, like the trends in the inflammatory markers, such as my C-reactive protein (CRP) and white blood cell count, and the rate at which they were coming down.

I know I found it very stressful that everyone was concentrating solely on numbers on a chart, or what drug dosage needed to be altered to address whichever problem. For the first week, nobody would comment on whether I was looking or getting any better, and I increasingly felt like it was up to me to determine whether I was improving because everyone was fixated on the measurable results.

I was especially concerned about improvement because, even from my very first days in the ward, I was obsessed with being allowed to go home. One time I got very upset because I had a temperature of 38.2 degrees and was shivering under my blanket in layers of sweaters. The 'Bond girl' nurse ordered me to sit up in bed and remove my layers of clothing while she opened the window. I got very upset and started crying, partly because I was freezing (though it was admittedly very warm in the room), but mostly because I was worried that this episode was somehow going to impede my release date. When Trevor came in and saw me in tears, sitting by an open window, he went and confronted the nurse – Scrappy-Doo style – and strongly suggested that she deal with the situation more sensitively. She defended her position, but what reassured me most was that Trevor said that she would have no power to make decisions, only to record what she had observed.

I'm fortunate that the majority of nurses and doctors on the ward were very helpful and compassionate. When you're already feeling that weak and vulnerable, a few kind words go a long way. As there were different people appearing every day, I was pleased when I saw familiar faces, especially among the nurses. It was hard to build up a rapport with most, as there were so many. Sometimes I mixed some of them up, especially as they all wore the same royal blue nurses' uniform, though at least the health care workers wore grey, which helped distinguish who to speak to about what.

But some of the staff I got to know pretty well, and they were nearly all very kind to me, patient and attentive. Most of them didn't know my whole story (other than what they had read in the medical charts), but a few had remembered me from the first surgery and wondered what had happened to me. They recognised me, but of course I didn't recognise them. All of them were horrified to hear what had happened to me, claiming they'd never seen anything like that occur on their ward.

Whether they were touched by my story or it was their nature, some of the nurses and health care workers became quite fond of me and tried to relate to me more as a person, and would do whatever they could to help, whether it was in their exact remit or not. Some shared details of their lives, which I appreciated, especially since my own life had been virtually decimated at that point. One of the health care workers, Pat, would visit regularly and chat freely about her life. She was very interested in what I ate, and I eventually got Trevor to bring her a recipe for one of my favourite vegan quiches. One night nurse stands out in my mind. In her spare time, she constructed and baked elaborate cakes. She told me about a Minecraft cake she was making for her son's birthday. A few weeks later I saw her again and she showed me incredible photos of it on her phone.

The days passed without any kind of fixed routine, other than my medications being administered at certain times of the day and night, and nurses would always try to keep to that schedule as much as possible. They also came as quickly as they could when I rang the call button. Of course, sometimes the ward could be quite busy. I wouldn't have had any real awareness of this in my 'bubble' of a room. Often a nurse would say, 'I'll be back in a minute,' and I wouldn't see her for another four hours, or sometimes not at all if she got drawn in elsewhere. I would often ask them if they were having a busy night, only to hear of all the emergencies being brought in or ladies with diabetes who needed tending at 3 a.m.

As I said, I never heard or was aware of much from my room. A couple of nights there were police roaming the ward but nothing was ever explained, despite my commenting on it, so presumably the staff were told not to say anything about it. Some weekends the ward was on 'intake duty', whereby every emergency from anywhere would be sent to the tiny Hawthorn Ward and it was manically busy. It probably also explained why some nights there were men roaming around a gynaecological ward. But it also meant that nurses would sometimes take an extremely long time to get to me to give me my nightly medication, which I had to wait for before I could attempt to drift off to sleep.

One strange consequence of compiling this account from my notes, and supplemented with the detailed medical records, is how many events happened on different days or at different times than I had remembered. For example, several incidents may have happened on one single day that I thought had occurred on different days. I guess it's because days can seem very long in hospital when you're stationary in one place, and the only stimulus is derived from people coming in and out. Thinking about it now, it was sort of a relief it was in the summer, because at least when it started to get dark I knew it was evening – around 8.30 p.m. If it had been winter and getting dark at 4 p.m., I would have had virtually no sense of time passing.

One of the worst things about being in hospital is all of the waiting around…waiting to hear results, waiting to hear what the plan is, then being told what the plan is, only to be told via another nurse that it's now a different plan…waiting for the 'back in a minute' and several hours would go by. All these things were so stressful and not conducive to healing. I don't know if hospital time forces you to be patient, or just succeeds in wearing you down.

From my two weeks in intensive care, I had learned the valuable lesson about how precious life is, and yet I found myself bored and restless, willing the hours to go by, thinking only in terms of what time the consultant would be coming or that Trev would be back with my dinner in an hour's time.

When I think about how much I would usually accomplish in a day, it drove me crazy watching the hours go by, waiting, waiting, waiting. Ironically, I say I was watching the hours go by, but literally I wasn't because the clock ticking in the room was wrecking my head so Trevor kindly climbed up and disabled it, putting the battery in backwards. The best part about this (apart from there being no annoying ticking noises) was that every single person that came in – especially the nurses doing my obs, who needed to record the time… If they didn't have a nurse's watch, they would look at the clock and say, 'Oh, that's not working. Do you have the time?' Nobody thought it strange that the clock wasn't working, and not one person the whole time I was there suggested fixing it or replacing the battery – thank goodness.

NOURISHMENT

Trevor sorting out the clock was one of innumerable ways he helped and looked after me. I increasingly relied on Trevor to do almost everything for me. He was my shopper and chef, my advocate and hero, as well as my only source of contact other than the doctors and hospital staff.

While I communicated with my friends via texts and occasional emails on Trevor's phone (there was no functioning Wi-Fi on this ward either), I absolutely did not want anyone to come and visit me. I was ashamed of what had happened to me and embarrassed about the state I was in and how I looked. Plus, I didn't have much of an attention span, and wasn't feeling charitable enough to hear about how great other people's summers had been and where they had been on holiday. I didn't end up seeing any friends until a month after this whole sorry business had begun, though I very much appreciated the cards and good wishes, among which was a small knitted owl sent by a friend in Canada.

So, the only company I allowed was Trevor, who was steadfast and unwavering in his presence. I'm extremely lucky to have had Trevor throughout this entire ordeal, and perhaps even luckier that it happened in August when he was free and not teaching much (though it messed up any other plans he might have had, such as going out busking every day).

There aren't words adequate to describe the tremendous help and support he was through it all. Trevor was with me in that small room in the hospital every single day, sometimes the whole day and into the evening. He had a (fairly uncomfortable) chair opposite the bed, in which he would be content to sit for hours, often working on things on his phone, or interacting with all the medical team that came into my room. I'm sure I wasn't great company for him, though I was immensely grateful for his. He literally could not do enough for me, cycling backwards and forwards, schlepping food, clothes and various personal items, re-arranging his entire days around keeping me and our household going.

Our relationship and the significant part he played in my recovery added another somewhat unique element to the whole situation. As mentioned, Trevor and I have been close friends for almost fifteen years, and in a relationship for many of them. The past three years we've been just friends, albeit best friends, and we still live together in the same house.

During the previous year, we'd been going through particular challenges in our relationship, but when the time of my surgery came round, Trevor agreed to be available and also to act as my partner, especially in the unlikely event (so we thought) of there being a need to consult with a next of kin. Little did we know how long this charade would go on for, and how invaluable it would end up being in enabling Trevor to be so involved in the course of my treatment.

Of course, my becoming critically ill had the unsurprising effect of cutting through our previous problems and bringing us closer together again – as friends, but we maintained the pretence of being in a relationship because it enabled Trevor to continue to play an active role in the decision making regarding my care.

Though I dislike being dishonest, even when I rejoined the land of the living, it just seemed easier to let the medical team assume we were partners, if not actually married, such that even when they referred to Trevor as my husband I didn't bother correcting them. The only time I did was when a doctor I'd never seen before addressed me as 'Mrs Lavine' and referred to Trevor as 'Mr Lavine'. That was just too weird, and I suggested he just call us Trevor and Kirsten, as did most of the staff who got to know us.

I think people were generally touched by Trevor's unwavering loyalty, and a few wanted to know where we had met and how long we'd been together. Certainly everyone got used to seeing Trevor as a regular fixture on the ward. Although there were supposedly set visiting hours (a couple of hours in the afternoon and evening), whether it was because I was such a special case or because Trevor was bringing me all of my food, he was increasingly allowed to be there at all hours, and nobody said anything if he was still with me sometimes until well past 10 p.m.

Food was another pressing issue. After my one initial attempt at a limp lettuce and tomato salad (which Trevor probably ended up eating), I never again tried to order anything from the hospital menu. There was nothing vegan anyway, and from what I saw, I was amazed that anyone was expected to get better eating any of it. (Even the water tasted terrible for some reason, and I only drank the water Trevor brought from home or from the water coolers in the main building.) So the staff were remarkably accommodating about Trevor bringing me my meals, and at any time he chose to do so. Some were even interested in the particulars of what he'd made.

But poor Trevor. It's a wonder he didn't end up in the psychiatric ward with all the hassle that feeding me brought. In short, I was having serious issues eating. At first I found it hard to eat anything. Bizarrely, I was actually able to eat more in the ICU. Perhaps my body hadn't had time to realise what state I was in then, and was instinctually trying to revert back to how I was eating before. By the time I got to Hawthorn Ward, for whatever reason, I simply wasn't able to eat very much. I still had a dietician harping on about the need for more protein intake, but not as severely as in the ICU, so I could relax a bit and just eat whatever I was able to – which wasn't much.

At first I seemed okay with sweet things like fruit and plain soya yogurt with jam. I also drank a lot of protein shakes, which placated the hospital staff and seemed to do me some good. Trevor continued making me smoothies with blueberries, bananas, spinach, barley grass and spirulina, which I seemed to be able to ingest. Most of the time I wasn't hungry, and would force myself to drink these protein shakes and smoothies which, along with two iron multivitamins a day, were basically keeping me alive.

In the beginning, I could also eat a bit of soup, but then *Salt-mageddon* kicked in. Simply put, everything, and I mean *everything* I tried tasted too salty. Though I never fully got an answer to this, I put it down to the antibiotics I was on. Later on, I read an excellent booklet put out by the hospital's ICU department, and one of the things it stated was how your taste buds can be affected and that food, for example, may end up tasting salty. It was odd but everything I put in my mouth, from cereal to plain oatcakes and even plain soup, tasted unbearably salty.

Even when I was hungry it was hard for me to eat because everything tasted so strange. Sweet things were about the only thing I could manage. Trevor often brought me fruit salads he had lovingly prepared, and I would attempt to eat a bit before handing the rest over to him. (Trevor ate a helluva lot of fruit that month, especially melon and pineapple which wouldn't keep long in the fridge.) I drank a lot of grape juice and, as mentioned, plain soya yogurt was one of the few things I could eat consistently, and I scoffed it like there was no tomorrow. This is possibly because of the probiotic cultures it contained, which perhaps I instinctually knew I needed to counter all of the antibiotics that were making my digestion worse and worse. (Eventually I got given a probiotic and, incredibly, an entire bottle to take home when I was discharged.)

But I continued to have a problem eating solid food for several weeks. For those who think vegans are limited in what they eat, I really learned how limiting it was to be on a solely watery or sweet liquid diet. And I wasn't getting any stronger on it either. Later on, I could sometimes manage half an avocado and a small bowl of oat cereal which had been soaked in rice milk for an hour. A week later I started to eat corn pasta with plain tomato passata. I'd manage about a quarter of a bowl for dinner and this was a real triumph for me. I even began to look forward to it.

SLEEPING AND CONCENTRATION

Sleeping was another ongoing challenge in hospital. It was almost impossible for me to sleep at night, and I don't remember a single night where I slept other than in small snatches of an hour or two at a time. There were many reasons for my problems sleeping. For starters, I wasn't in great shape. In the beginning my lungs were filled with residual water from all the IV fluids, and I was coughing a lot, especially at night. I had a cannula with two tubes attached to the back of my hand, which was very obtrusive, and I also had to sleep in embolic stockings, which were tight and made me feel too warm. Once I started wearing my own clothes, I could at least sleep in jogging bottoms and a T-shirt, which was more comfortable than the hospital gown.

Then there was all the medication I was on, some of which had to be administered at night. Come 9 p.m., I would start getting anxious thinking about the nightly round of medication, which would usually appear sometime between 10–11 p.m. The worst aspect was the Clexane injection, which I would ask to be done first to get it over with. This was to treat the blood clot I'd obtained in my leg and consisted of a sharp injection in my stomach. Every night a nurse would glance in dismay at my abdomen covered in scars and look for somewhere to put the injection that wouldn't aggravate the existing sores. Although the nurses were gentle and very caring, the injection was incredibly painful (like a horrible piercing in the stomach), and it would take a full fifteen minutes for the pain to subside.

Then there were the antibiotics. Some I took orally, but generally I had some sort of IV which every night had to drip through two bags, which took twenty minutes each. I was hooked up to a machine, so I couldn't move or go anywhere until the bags were finished draining. Then I was put on another antibiotic that took over an hour to drip through. The odd time when I had to go to the loo during its administration, I had to take the machine with me. It was difficult sitting in bed, tired but not able to sleep, until the IV had finished dripping. I remember I used to play Quadra Pop on my (ancient) phone, or occasionally I typed up notes for this account on my computer.

And then, as mentioned earlier, there was the waiting for a nurse to come. I often urged Trev to leave before 10 p.m. because it would be getting really dark outside (and he had no bike lights), and sometimes I wouldn't be hooked up to the machine until 10.30 p.m., and it often wouldn't finish until well after 11 p.m. Since the ward woke up by 6 a.m., I was never likely to get a full night's sleep, even if I had been able to.

Of course, my own general state of health didn't help matters. My temperature fluctuated all the time, either from the infection or all the antibiotics, so I was often too hot and then too cold. The room was always very stuffy, though I could open the windows, which helped a bit. Mercifully, as well as having the privacy of my own room, I had my own bathroom, which was a godsend as I was often up going to the loo in the middle of the night.

Noise from the ward was sometimes a problem, though not as much as it could have been, but the lights from the hallway shone very brightly into the room. It was usually around 11 p.m. that they were eventually turned off. Of course, I was often not very tired, since I was immobile most of the day and usually slept in short spurts throughout the day. So at night I would lie in bed cuddling Chubb Chubb and Bonnie, a plush puppy, and play soothing music all night on a portable CD player, though the batteries kept conking out. It was awful, lying there all night feeling hot or cold, helpless and frustrated, silently willing the morning to arrive faster. I considered it a real achievement if I could sleep for a whole hour or two, which was often just before dawn. I knew it wouldn't be long before the ward sprang into action at 6 a.m., if not before.

It always surprised me how early the nursing staff would come around in the morning. You would think that unless a patient rang the call button, it would have been best to leave them to get some much-needed sleep. The first to arrive were usually health care workers, bringing round jugs of water about 5.45 a.m. I eventually got them to stop doing that by showing them all of the bottles of water Trevor kept me well stocked with. One time I was fast asleep at 5.30 a.m. when a nurse came round to check on me and succeeded in waking me up, for which she was very apologetic. Eventually, I decided it was less stressful for me to simply be up with the birds as soon as it got light, around 5.30 a.m., and open the blinds and declare myself awake, so as not to be woken up by the rounds which began in earnest at 6 a.m.

Once I became aware of the early starts and how little time I would have to myself before the daily rounds of medical visits began, I decided to begin my day the way I used to in my 'normal' life. I couldn't go outside and feed the birds or do my morning stretches, but I could sit up and try to meditate for a bit, which is how I always began each morning. Once the health care workers stopped offering me breakfast, since they knew Trevor was bringing me food, I could have a bit of free time between 6–7 a.m. So I would meditate as best I could for about fifteen minutes, and then read some affirmations and prayers.

Then I would text Trevor to say I was up and he would usually call me. I should say it here, since I haven't said it elsewhere, and since I'm discussing spiritual matters: For reasons completely unknown to me, whenever Trevor called, the entire screen on my phone would light up blue. It still does this and only with

Trevor calling and nobody else. If anyone out there in the old mobile phone industry can shed light on this, I would be very interested to know the reason.

So Trev and I would have a chat, and I would list what I wanted him to bring that day and what I was likely to be able to eat. Then I would begin the morning struggle of figuring out how to get up, wash and change my clothes. In the first few days, when I was really exhausted, I often wouldn't accomplish this until late morning.

After the first day's disaster in the sit-down shower in the hallway, I decided to try and use my own en-suite shower. By the third day I could stand for a few minutes, but had the problem of keeping the cannula on my hand dry, so one arm was covered in a plastic bag, rendering it unusable. The shower was in an awkward triangular shape and the shower head was so hard to manoeuvre that I kept flooding the bathroom floor. With Trevor's help, I persisted, though it was a process that I never quite got right.

I suppose I could have just stayed in my same clothes and not bothered washing or changing. But other than the fact that I still had some uterine bleeding, given that I was obsessed with going home, I felt I had to demonstrate that I could perform normal tasks like washing, dressing and changing my clothes each day, even if I was only in shlumpy jogging gear. I always needed Trevor's help putting on the embolic stockings, which I had to wear every day, since if I put them on wrongly, they would supposedly do more harm than good.

Other than Trevor's company, there wasn't a lot of stimulation. I had a portable radio I kept tuned to Classic FM, as much for the soothing music as to hear news bulletins from the 'outside world'. Another one of my pastimes was picking off all of the bits of rubber medical tape from my neck and chest, guided by a hand mirror. I discovered that soap and water did nothing to dislodge them and, as mentioned, my entire front was covered with them, so it took a long time to get rid of it all.

Once I had settled into the ward, it dawned on me that I should be taking some notes for posterity. Trevor had already printed off the detailed daily diary he had written while I was in the ICU, which I read with a combination of fascination, horror and sadness. I remember feeling incredibly moved by everything he had done for me, especially while I was unconscious, and it made me cry continuously. I kept feeling shocked at what had happened to the main character, then having to remind myself that I was the main character, as it all seemed so unreal to me.

I thought I ought to begin to record my own experiences, and I now had my little laptop to do so. The problem was one of concentration. Also, for the first week, I had a cannula on the back of my hand, which made typing difficult, as it kept banging against the keys. When they eventually changed it, I asked that it be put further up so I could have better use of my hand and keep my fingers free.

One of the first things I'd said in my notes was how I wished I could have started writing sooner or written more at the time. Usually I could manage about half an hour in the morning before the assault course of people began. This was when my mind was clearest and I could attempt to focus.

Though I am normally quite a voracious reader, I found reading about other subjects virtually impossible. I was so weak and unfocused that I found it extremely difficult to concentrate to any degree. Books were impossible, as I simply couldn't focus on the story, and ultimately didn't care about the plight of anyone else at that time. Eventually I could glance at the local newspaper, and one day Trevor came back armed with a wide variety of magazines on fashion, health, nature, walking and history. Not knowing what to buy me, he generously bought me several of each. I attempted to get through these and they kept me going for a while.

Ultimately, though, between medical visits, I had nothing to do, and was incredibly frustrated and restless. One of the main problems was that there was nowhere to go in the ward, and no one really to talk to. In fairness, they did have a 'day room', a rather cheerless place with a patient fridge, vending machines, a TV and unappealing magazines and books. I tried going there a few times, as much for the achievement of walking the 50 feet down the corridor as for a change of scenery, but I just found it too depressing. No one sat in there and socialised. Very occasionally there was somebody watching TV (I don't watch TV so this never appealed to me), but no one sat at the tables and had coffee or anything like that. I tried eating there a few times just to get out of the habit of eating in my bed, but I just found it too depressing and preferred to eat in my room, where at least I could talk to Trevor in privacy.

But the problem was that I literally felt trapped in the room – feeling trapped being one of my worst nightmares. I felt trapped with nothing to do, short of waiting for a nurse or doctor to come and having no idea when they were going to appear. 'Normality' became a series of blood tests and medications, so much so that the outside world just disappeared. Trevor would describe going to the shop to buy food and I'd think this was nirvana – something so completely beyond my reach. I was thoroughly obsessed with getting out and going home.

I guess this was partly because this was an unplanned stay in hospital and I hadn't blocked out the mental space for it. Also, because I was unconscious or delirious during the worst of the infection's hold on me, I was never able to appreciate the gravity of the calamity that befell me or the magnitude of what was wrong with me. Most days I just felt unwell, and I attributed my weakened state, my pain, my hot sweats and inability to eat as much to the side effects of the medications as to being in hospital in general.

I felt, even from my time in intensive care, that whatever was wrong with me I could deal with better at home, in my own space. Going home became my sole ambition. Never mind the fact that I had spent the last year trying to get out of the house, where I felt I spent too much time and which was getting me down. Now that I had not been home for nearly a month, it was the one thing I wanted more than anything.

Much later, a consultant would write in a report about it being 'a very frightening time for me' but actually, I don't really remember ever feeling scared. This was my only fear – that as one day rolled into the next without any change, and with nobody telling me when I would be going home, that I would be stuck there forever and never be allowed out.

But most of all, I couldn't accept that my life, as I knew it, had effectively been cancelled, and I'd been placed in this surreal parallel universe. Although I was somewhat in a state of limbo with regards to many aspects of my life, I still hadn't accepted all the things I had missed or would be missing in future. Quite apart from losing any freelance and temporary work, that month saw a big outdoor fiesta roll by, an ignored invitation to a friend's family in Italy, a cancelled visit from Trevor's sister and brother-in-law in the Midlands, a puppetry festival where I was due to volunteer… I often wonder where I would be now if I had fulfilled many of the things in my diary.

ON THE MOVE

At least I regained my mobility fairly early on. The whole ordeal would have been so much worse if I'd not been able to move. I gather from Mr Ellis's astonishment on my first day in the ward, seeing me ambling about with the walker, that this isn't the usual trajectory for people newly released from intensive care. After two days, I decided I didn't need the walker anymore and just started walking (slowly) without it.

One of the things I'm strangely proud of is that I never once fell in hospital. I was always very careful and extremely mindful of my own state of weakness. Having said that, I remember once walking to the day room with something to put in the under-counter fridge. I had to squat to reach it, and then I couldn't get up again, as I didn't have any muscle strength in my legs. I remained motionless for a few minutes until I eventually had the presence of mind to pull over a chair and push myself up that way.

The coming days would provide further tests of my mobility and endurance. One of the first tastes of freedom I had was when I was allowed to leave the ward building in a wheelchair and go with Trevor on a little jaunt. Up until that point, I had only ever been transported to and from the main building by ambulance, and so it had essentially been about two and a half weeks since I had been outside for some fresh air.

The feeling was absolutely blissful. Trevor wheeled me the five minutes it took to get to the main building. I had a look in the shop (surprisingly terrible – I was barely able to get a newspaper), and I practised walking a bit between seating areas, setting goals for myself to get from one seating area to the other. I would tire very easily and not be able to walk very much. But with each outing, I attempted to walk a little bit more. One day it rained, but so as not to miss our outing, Trevor simply bundled me up and I held up an umbrella and kept dry (though he probably got soaked) as we made our way to the main building.

I enjoyed being wheeled around in my 'chariot', as Trevor called it, though being hospital grounds, there weren't many places to go other than to the main building. However, we did go to a parkette across the road from my ward. On sunny days, I could sit on a bench with Trevor and enjoy the flowers and the birds singing and people eating their lunch. It was hard for me to sit up for very long, and I remember one time lying down on a bench with my head on Trevor's lap and dozing in the sunshine.

On the fifth day in the ward, I was permitted to go home for a few hours. After receiving my afternoon IV antibiotics, I was allowed out and didn't have to come back until 9 p.m. that evening, for the next round of medication. It felt like I had finally been let out of prison. I hadn't seen my house for so long, and it felt very, very odd to go inside. The stairs, which had always seemed steep, were especially a challenge. To go upstairs I had to pull myself up holding on to the banister, and to get down I had to descend on my bum. But it was so wonderful to see my room at long last, and when I sank down into my bed for the first time I nearly cried as I finally felt safe in my own room again.

I spent much of my first afternoon sleeping peacefully, enjoying the quiet, and then I attempted to use the shower. Although it was a big step up into the bathtub, I just knew instinctually that, even with a plastic bag still wrapped around one arm, I would find it easier to use my own shower that I was familiar with. And so I had my first real, proper shower in over three weeks, and I could finally get dressed without worrying about anyone barging in on me.

The next day I was once again allowed to go home in the afternoon. We had to wait for the IV antibiotics to finish dripping through and for the nurse to remove the tube from the IV bag. I'm not sure if she was running late or it just took an incredibly long time for the antibiotic to drip through, but I remember getting stressed because Trevor had a ukulele group to teach in the east of the city, and if we didn't leave soon he was going to be late for it (which is, indeed, what happened). I felt terrible about this. I had already disrupted enough of his life that month and didn't want to cause any further upset.

Because of how late he was, he ended up having to drop me off at home and dash off. It was the first time I was left on my own, and even though I was at home, in my own bed, I was still quite scared in case anything happened. This is how far I had fallen, that I was afraid to be left completely alone. I remember lying in bed, trying but being unable to sleep and checking the time every half hour. I was relieved when Trevor returned. I felt safe with him there by my side, looking after my every need in this strange, new world.

This became my routine for the next few days. I woke up at 5.30 a.m. and stayed in hospital till the afternoon, and then was 'let out' for a few hours, promising to return by 9 p.m. for my nightly medication, followed by an overnight stay in hospital. It was incredible how flexible the medical team were and I was pleasantly surprised. It was also fortunate that we only lived a seven-minute drive from the hospital. It was pretty much around the corner from us, one of the things I found so ironic, that this whole dramatic episode literally occurred on our doorstep.

This 'day release' meant that every afternoon I could have a shower and sleep undisturbed for a couple of hours in the comfort and safety of my own bed. I would get up around

6 p.m., once Trevor had prepared 'dinner'. This was another round of experiments, since I still had trouble eating most foods, but we eventually settled on me eating a quarter bowl of corn pasta and plain tomato sauce, which is what I ate every single night and, as mentioned, I even started to look forward to it and enjoy it. And, as always, I had soya yogurt for dessert – my one consistent food. Then I would lie on the sofa and feel anxious, watching the time get closer for when we had to return to hospital. At 8.50 p.m., I would reluctantly get up and slip on my pink Crocs, which I wore everywhere, and we would proceed back to hospital.

A few days later, an even greater event occurred: I was allowed to sleep at home – all night! This was truly a blissful watershed. I'll never forget my first night at home. It was so quiet, so dark, so peaceful. Trevor slept with the door to his room open in case I needed anything. On this and subsequent nights, I finally had the experience again of being able to sleep properly, sometimes nearly a whole night. Trevor, on the other hand, probably didn't get much sleep at all throughout this whole period.

Although I was definitely sleeping more, I still woke up every morning with a terrible stomach ache, headache and was usually sweaty all over. Most mornings I wouldn't venture out of bed without first taking ibuprofen, and even then it took a long, long time for me to get up, and the stomach aches and sweatiness rarely abated. These, I assume, were a result of the antibiotics I was being given at night at hospital.

After I'd managed to get up, I'd have to return to the hospital in the morning for the team to assess where I was at. At this stage my inflammatory CRP level was going down, though it was still over 100 (normal being 7), and my heart rate was still very high. I would spend all morning waiting for various people to appear – the nurses to administer antibiotics and compile observations, as well as having a brief exchange with the consultant on his or her rounds.

The best time for me became the afternoons, when I was allowed out of hospital and went home. I was still very weak and so rarely ventured too far from the house. Sometimes I would ask Trevor to let me off a few houses down from ours, and I would walk the rest of the way home – thoroughly shattered when I got there. Another time, I was desperate to go for a walk and be in nature, and we ventured out to a particular place along the river because it was flat. I walked probably half a mile – slowly – taking breaks sitting on benches. It was a huge achievement for me but also very exhausting.

I'd carry on with my afternoon routine of resting and trying to eat, and then we'd go back to the hospital every night at 9 p.m., for a supposedly quick round of antibiotics and other medication. And every night for one reason or another – the nurses being short-staffed or busy or dealing with emergencies – the whole process of waiting and administrating the medication would take two hours, and I would get home at 11 p.m., exhausted and overwrought.

There was one particularly stressful incident one night. I needed a new cannula put in my hand (the painful procedure had to be carried out every few days to prevent infection). We waited an hour, whereupon a very young and rather smug doctor (the exception, it has to be said) came by to insert the new cannula. He made a number of inappropriate, unprofessional remarks and was very curt with me. I suggested the spot on my wrist where I preferred he put the cannula, but he was in a hurry and insisted on inserting it in the big vein in the crook of my arm. It was a terrible place to put it, and every time I bent my arm to do anything I would feel the needle shooting through me. I was too upset to think straight, but fortunately Trevor had the presence of mind to realise this needed to be remedied, and at almost midnight we drove back to the hospital and got someone to take it out for me. Thank God, or it would have been agony.

By this stage I was back in touch with my friends, and two of my closest friends wanted to come and visit me at home. I told them about my 'schedule', and they agreed to come one afternoon after they had finished work. They turned up with a beautiful hanging plant, and looked tanned and happy from their holidays in Italy. I felt okay, but was still very tired and had to lie on the sofa while I talked to them. I think they were both shocked by my appearance and even more by my crazy story. I was happy that things were going well in their lives. One of them was off to Krakow that weekend, so I dug out my guidebook on the city and some zlotys left over from my time spent living there, and gave them to her to take with on her trip.

During their visit, Sandra, the consultant, called Trevor. She asked for me but thought I might be sleeping. 'No,' he said, 'she's entertaining!' It seems as if we were forever surprising them. Sandra called to say that she had been in contact with a radiologist, who had agreed to carry out an image-guided drainage procedure, and which was most likely going to take place the very next day, Friday. This was highly unusual, as the radiologist usually performed such surgeries on Wednesdays, but she'd insisted that this couldn't wait, and basically pulled out all the stops to get him to agree to do it in the first place, and the next day at that. I don't think I appreciated at the time how incredible this action was. Neither Trevor nor I knew much about what this procedure entailed, but since it was something that offered the promise of my situation improving somewhat, we went forward in faith.

The next morning at 11 a.m., I returned to the hospital for another surgical procedure – nearly a month since the original one – and I spent most of the day waiting for it to occur. I wasn't looking forward to more surgery but my options were limited. I wrote at the time that I couldn't take much more of my situation. I remember that I wasn't able to eat or drink all day and it was a very long and stressful wait.

At some point during the day a junior doctor, who was new to me, came in and asked – out of the blue – how I'd feel about having a blood transfusion, and would it be against my beliefs. I felt quite weird about the whole idea but we found out later that I'd already had one anyway, weeks before in the ICU, and nobody had ever asked me (or Trevor) about it then. Apparently, despite my efforts in taking iron supplements, it was discovered the day before that my haemoglobin had dropped to 67, while a normal rate was 115–160, which I was required to have in order undergo surgery – hence the need for a blood transfusion.

Finally, at 4.45 p.m., I was transferred to the main building for the drainage procedure. Trev came with me by ambulance. We had a new nurse ride with us as an 'escort', who spent the whole trip with her eyes closed. I guess her role was more to escort my increasingly bulging medical file, which she held on to tightly while she seemingly dozed on the journey.

When I was being prepared for surgery, the radiologist came by, followed by Sandra, and a very strange conversation ensued. The radiologist went through very clearly and succinctly what the drainage procedure would entail, while expressing quite plainly that the likelihood of it working was actually very slim. I later discovered just how reluctant he was to perform this procedure, and how hard Sandra had worked to convince him to do it. He basically felt it was a waste of time, and that I would probably need a full pelvic clearance at some point anyhow to get rid of the reservoirs of infection that lay out of reach.

Despite Sandra's initial support for me going through with this procedure, she too must have lost faith in its effectiveness, because while I was waiting for the procedure to happen, she began to sow seeds of doubt in me and I got very confused and upset. It was only Trevor's unwavering presence of mind that said, 'Let's give this a go,' because he had a good feeling about it, which enabled it to go ahead. Thank goodness he did, because remarkably, and against anyone's expectations – it worked.

The procedure consisted of introducing into my cervix two thin probes about 3mm wide with small locking 'pigtail' swirls on the end, and with state-of-the-art imaging equipment, expertly steering these tubes into either side of my pelvis to reach the large reservoirs of infection, with the intention of draining and flushing out these last pockets of resistance. Afterwards, there would be two drains left attached for a few days to allow the flow to drain from the infected areas. Another drain went through my abdomen with a similar aim.

According to Trevor, the surgery took about two hours. When I awoke around 8 p.m. I had two drains coming out of my private parts and another from my abdomen draining into large plastic bags. The procedure resulted in draining almost a litre of pus-filled fluid, and apparently the anaesthetist said that as soon as the procedure started, my heart rate – which had been very high – began to go down. The bags, which had been emptied following the surgery, needed to be left attached for a couple of days to see if any more pus drained out. With these heavy bags and tubes and clips pulling on my bits it was all pretty sore, so I had to have a constant supply of painkillers, and it was a difficult night's sleep.

The next afternoon, after sitting in bed all morning with these huge bags, fortunately I was able to switch to 'leg bags', which could be strapped to my legs and at least allow me to be mobile. The bag from my abdomen was tucked into a flowery cloth bag, thanks to the cleverness of one of the nurses. Lots more painkillers ensued. With these tubes descending from my private parts, it was extremely awkward to walk around or to use the bathroom.

On Sunday morning, since the abdominal drain had hardly produced any pus (without any expectation that it would), it was agreed that it could be removed. A nurse came along and essentially yanked it out. It didn't really bother me since I was used to pain in that region for one reason or another, but Trevor was beside himself with distress. He was convinced that it was the way in which this drain was removed that was causing me whatever abdominal pain I had afterwards, and it took a long time and convincing from several sources to persuade him otherwise.

This was the last Sunday in August, and the final weekend of a summer-long display of sculptures which had been decorated according to different themes and dotted about town, their locations marked on an accompanying trail map. I had planned to spend much of August seeing them at my leisure, and now suddenly I had only one day to see any of them at all. Bags strapped to me or not, I was determined to go and see them. Trev was incredibly obliging.

So there I was, in joggers and no underwear (which was impossible to put on) with the bottom cuffs of the joggers (hopefully) covering the two leg drainage bags. On a map Trevor had brought to the hospital, I circled the sculptures I really wanted to see, and Trev drove as near to them as he could get and stayed in the car while I wobbled over to them to get a closer look. They were very good! There was one at the far side of a bridge that I wanted to see, so Trevor and I simply walked across the full length of the bridge and back. It took me a long time but I made it – no doubt bolstered by the blood transfusion which I'd received, which gave me a massive boost of energy. (A friend later joked that I looked so much better that I must have been given the blood of a twenty-year-old. Whoever you are – thank you very much, donor.)

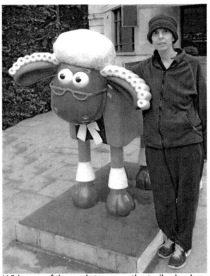

With one of the sculptures on the trail, a leg bag protruding from my calf, and wearing a fleece and a winter hat.

Two days after the surgical procedure very little else drained out into the bags, which suggested that most came out at the time of the surgery. Mr Ellis wanted to keep the drains in for another day, but Trev and I pleaded a convincing case that nothing would be gained by this, and so he agreed to take them out – thank goodness.

Everyone prayed that this procedure had done the job. My CRP on Sunday 30 August was 43, the first time it had been under 100 since the initial diagnosis. I wrote at the time: 'I certainly feel much better, but of course it will depend on what the markers say. So far my obs are much better than they were a week ago and I feel like I'm getting better.'

RELEASE AND RETURN TO HOSPITAL

My 'markers' were continuing to move in the right direction. After the Sunday, when my CRP level was down to 43, on Tuesday it was down again to 23. The results were so positive that it was decided to discharge me for good, once I was switched over to oral versions of the antibiotics. I also had to wait for someone qualified to take out my 'PICC line', which was a very long cannula (and one ultimately less vulnerable to infection), which had been put in during the drainage procedure to administer antibiotics. This was one of the last things that happened on the ward.

Part of the condition for my discharge was switching my IV antibiotic intake to tablets I could take myself. I remember waiting most of the day in hospital on the Thursday, while various antibiotics were chased up at the hospital pharmacy. I didn't like to stop and think what my treatment must have cost overall, but the NHS had decided at least to make the cost of the medication transparent by affixing a label on each packet with the price of the medication, should one need to refill it. I therefore knew how crazily expensive each of the medications were.

I was given a significant quantity of five different medications. Two of them, co-trimoxazole and metronidazole, were the antibiotics which I had to take two and three times a day respectively. I was also given a drug to help with the nausea caused by the antibiotics, along with an anti-spasmodic medication to help my stomach, to be used when required.

Added to this was the rivaroxaban I had to take twice a day for my blood clot. While I was immensely relieved to be free of the stabbing Clexane injections, my main concern about it was that I wasn't allowed to take ibuprofen while on rivaroxaban, but there was no way on earth I could survive my period (soon due) without ibuprofen. I was later told I could take ibuprofen sparingly, which is what I did.

I was officially discharged later that day, 3 September. Though relieved to finally be home for good, I felt overwhelmed and uneasy about all the medication I'd been charged with, and my days seemed to revolve around when I would be taking what. I felt especially negative towards the antibiotics and sensed strongly that my body didn't really want them. Since I had already vomited after taking these new ones for the first time, I was given an anti-nauseous drug to take with them, as well as an anti-spasmodic drug to act as a stomach muscle relaxant.

So I was taking these antibiotics and then being in horrible stomach pain lying on the bed, with nothing providing relief. We thought at the time that it was the antibiotics causing the pain. I knew that my system just didn't want to take them, and the first weekend after I was discharged I decided, against better medical judgement, to go off of them.

I say against better judgement because everything we'd read and been told stated that one of the worst things you can do is to stop antibiotic treatment in the middle of the course, because should the infection reoccur, it makes the bacteria more resistant to the antibiotic and therefore more difficult to treat. But I simply couldn't take any more. So I decided to stop taking them, and then incredibly, on that same day, we got a call from one of the doctors saying that I could stop taking the antibiotics, as the results of my most recent blood test showed that everything was looking relatively normal.

The first week at home I mainly mooched around on the sofa or lay on a sun lounger in the garden, as it was actually warm enough to do so. One or two of my friends dropped by and I filled them in on the horrific tale. I remember my first real outing was on 13 September, for the Open Doors heritage weekend. Trev, another friend and I went to a castle a two-hour drive away. I remember how steep I found it going up to the castle and how long it took me to get there. But we walked around the majestic rooms and the quaint village, and although I had to rest a bit, I was okay.

That afternoon, Trev was due to sing with his choir in a park back home, so we beetled up the motorway, only to encounter an accident which delayed us even further. But we made it just after they had begun the performance and he duly slotted himself in. There was a huge potluck buffet of food, which the people from the neighbourhood had brought, and much of it was vegan. I remember tucking in with gusto. I was so hungry, and though I probably didn't eat that much, it felt like a feast. However, my eating was still pretty erratic at this point. I was still getting stomach aches regularly, but they didn't seem to be coming from the infection, and we didn't know what was causing them.

By this time, I had started doing some temporary agency work in offices because I hadn't had any income for a month. If it hadn't been for my mum, I would have been really sunk financially. So, a couple of weeks after I was discharged I accepted some reception work for three afternoons that week, from Wednesday to Friday.

On the Wednesday morning, Trev and I had arranged to go to the hospital to see Sandra, regarding my curtailing the rivaroxaban blood clot medication earlier than the prescribed three months. I remember that morning it took me an incredibly long time to get out of bed because I was in terrible pain. We called and said we would be late, and Sandra was very accommodating. Eventually we got there, and Sandra had arranged for the head of haematology to come and discuss the rivaroxaban use with me. It was negotiated that since I was once again active and less in danger of acquiring further clots, I could take the medication for a total of six weeks, which meant I only had a couple of weeks left, which was a relief. Although I was still feeling pretty rough, I was determined to get to work that afternoon, which I did, buffered with a regular stream of ibuprofen. Somehow I got through the afternoon, trying to sit as still as possible, so as not to disturb my stomach further.

Unfortunately, Thursday morning I was in agony. We called Sandra and she advised us to come straight to the hospital and for me to expect to have to stay there overnight. Again, it took me a long time to get going, and when I finally reached the hospital, I was once again put in my own room in Hawthorn Ward (a different and actually nicer one). As I was in a lot of pain and shivering and vomiting, I was hooked up to IV paracetamol all day. All this pain necessitated me staying two nights in hospital, which was an awful return, the first night with a drip of liquid attached to me all night. Poor Trevor had brought me all kinds of food for dinner which I was looking forward to eating, only to be told I had to be nil by mouth.

I remember phoning the employment agency on the Thursday morning, telling them I was ill and saying that I wasn't going to make it to work that afternoon or the next day. I prayed that they couldn't make out via any tell-tale noises that I was in hospital, or 'Doctor proceed to the ward!' type announcements, but fortunately they didn't seem to cotton on and were actually very sympathetic. I was booked all the following week at another place and assured them that since I would have the weekend to recover, I would be well enough to return to work the following week. That was me all over – desperate to get on with my life and be free of this incapacitating situation.

The Thursday and Friday passed by very slowly. On Friday afternoon I went for a CT scan, and the results showed that I had a blockage in my small bowel, as a result of all the scarring from the infection. Later that afternoon, a member of Trevor's choir unexpectedly came to visit me with her two young daughters, who were performing in a festival at the hospital. I was pretty horrified since I looked and felt like hell. It was a kind thought, but I've learned always to ask if someone in hospital wants visitors and not just to assume they do.

That night, Trevor and I waited and waited for the bowel surgeons to come and give their assessment, based on the CT scan. By midnight they still hadn't come, so I told Trevor to go home, as they clearly weren't coming till morning. So Trevor went home and I went to sleep, only to be woken up at 1.30 a.m. by a troop of people I'd never seen before barging into the room and flicking on the lights. This was the apparent bowel surgery team who, without preamble, or much care for the time of night or how disoriented I was, began firing off a round of questions. They were implying that more surgery would be needed to deal with the blockage and I basically requested that they leave me in peace.

Trev came back early in the morning and I filled him in on the night's activities. He was soon followed by Mr Ellis, who was amused to see all my bags packed and me sitting on the bed ready to go home. I told him I would have gone out the window but couldn't get it open wide enough. I was only half joking.

That morning, Trevor was performing with his choir at the hospital as part of their weekend festival. Although I was literally next door to the main building, I wasn't well enough to get to the performance, but apparently it went very well. They had all kinds of acts participating. I would've liked to have seen the wheelchair dancers, I must admit.

Once Trevor came back from his choir performance, we waited all morning for the bowel surgeons to reappear with their latest assessment. That afternoon, Trevor and I were due to run our long-standing monthly recorder group in a town a 45-minute drive away, and there was no way I was missing that. Trevor did the teaching and I only did the admin and served the tea and biscuits, but it was a commitment that I always tried to honour. In fact, owing to the recent round of being in hospital, I still hadn't had a chance to bake the homemade cookies I always prepared for the group. I was still planning on going home that morning and rustling up a batch of something.

The morning passed, time kept ticking on and there was no sign of the bowel surgeons. I kept asking the doctor on duty – a lovely Scottish woman – to keep chasing them, which she continued to attempt to do, but still they didn't come. I assured her that I was feeling much better and had fulfilled their stated criteria for my release, which was the nausea abating and me opening my bowels. I felt all I needed to do was to recover at home and pay close attention to what I was eating.

By noon – Trevor having already alerted the recorder group that we were going to be late – we announced to the hospital team that we had to go, and the Scottish doctor was able to at least get the bowel surgeons on the phone to authorise my release and get my discharge papers going. We left at 12.45 p.m. We raced home, and with Trevor's help, I threw together some raw chocolate balls and we whizzed up the motorway. We arrived at the session half an hour late. When we entered the room the whole group applauded, as everyone had been made aware of the dreadful circumstances. I remember dozing on the lawn all afternoon in between making tea for the group.

After that, it took another month before the small bowel blockage cleared up. I was very careful about what I ate and the quantities, though once I could start eating more and a greater variety of things, I found I was really hungry all the time and ate constantly. My goal was to be 'eating normally' by the time Trev and I went to the Isle of Wight for a weekend at the end of October to celebrate my return to the land of the living. I remember on the trip I ate ravenously. I would buy, for example, samosas to have for lunch, and by 9 a.m. I was tucking into them and suddenly they were all gone. So I was sort of out of control, but on the other hand, it gave me a huge appreciation for food and for being able to eat once again.

PART 4
AFTERWARDS

Recovery is a strange process. No one gives you a set time for how long things are going to take, or the order in which they will occur, and neither is it a linear process, but instead it is full of setbacks. I have also found recovering mentally and emotionally from this experience to be an even greater challenge. Physically, it's possible to see progress, however small. But the mind can be a harsh critic, and wounds of the soul can be very hard to mend.

But once I was finally home for good – and there was no way I was going back to hospital again – I worked on healing all aspects of myself. Physically, this meant resting for great periods of time, even though I was keen to get working and be active again. Psychologically, this meant coming to terms with what had happened to me, and trying to make sense of it all and to learn to move on from it in time.

Physical and health issues

Physical recovery has been an odd progression. It started with me being able to eat more and more. Then it was a case of building up my energy to walk more and to go further. I remember how exhausting it was initially just covering a short distance, followed by the joy of being able to walk greater distances, until I could walk wherever I wanted to, within reason. Trev and I were used to going for walks every weekend in the countryside, which included going up sloping, uneven paths. It was a slow process to do this again, and I was extremely gratified when I could once again walk up inclines of any kind.

I also remember the first time I got on my bicycle again. It was three weeks after Mr Ellis's comment about the likelihood of me being able to cycle in about six months' time. I was very nervous, as I wasn't sure what my balance would be like. In any case, I only went to the local shop, and was alright. I also cycled to my follow-up appointments with Sandra, which surprised her. But I didn't see the point of seeing myself as a victim, and anyway, it wasn't that far to the hospital.

It took quite a bit longer to build back all the muscle strength I had lost, especially in my arms. I had an adequate means of testing this because I'd been doing yoga-type stretches for many years now in the mornings, including sun salutations. Part of this involves pushing yourself up from a prone position towards standing in a 'downward dog' pose, with arms extended down in front of you. It took me a full three months before I had the strength to push myself up. It was a blissful moment when I was finally able to do it.

Even to this day, owing to the scarring and potential damage to my small bowel (the extent of which I am still trying to ascertain), I continue to have recurring issues with eating and digestion. This has resulted in additional restrictions on what I can eat and when, and has compounded the already challenging components of my endometriosis.

Other physical remnants from my time in the ICU include two round marks on my neck where tubes were, though fortunately, I was spared the more prominent tracheotomy scar across my neck. However, there are ugly, disfiguring scars all across my stomach, down my belly button, and on my abdomen and pelvis. Though they no longer itch all the time, nor are as bright red, they are still as prominent as ever, even after regularly applying all kinds of oils and creams.

If this weren't enough, three months after I came home, just as I thought I was well on the road to returning to normal, another nasty surprise awaited: my hair started falling out en masse. The first sign was when my lustrous, curly hair started thinning and going straight, and while brushing it one morning, I noticed clumps of it coming out, which happened on subsequent days until I simply stopped brushing it at all in an attempt to stem the tide. Apparently hair loss is a normal consequence of having had sepsis, and most medics seemed to think it would grow back in time. It took many more months before my hair started growing back at all and there's still not as much of it, though what there is has grown back healthier and in much tighter curls. All I can say is that it's been incredibly upsetting, and a blow to my self-esteem.

Another legacy of recovering from sepsis has been not knowing what long-term toll the infection and all the antibiotics are likely to have had on my system. For example, I am still very tired much of the time and, as mentioned, have chronic stomach problems and the occasional small bowel blockage, with its accompanying searing pain.

I continue to monitor my body's activities and pay close attention to what I eat, and try to supplement my diet with probiotic and gut-friendly foods, but nothing has completely solved these problems even to this day. I'm now a lot more sensitive to light and noise and, as my immune system took a serious battering, I seem to catch colds and viruses much more frequently than I used to.

An additional long-term impact is that I am now marked as someone that, having contracted a blood clot, is possibly more likely to get one again in the future. It has implications every time I consider a new medication, which may come with increased risks if you've had blood clots.

A greater issue is flying, especially long-haul flights. I've been instructed to wear embolic stockings, to ensure I walk and move around a lot on board, and most recently, was advised by a haematologist never to fall asleep on a flight. A tall order on an overnight flight from Canada!

The first flight I took was a few months after I came home from hospital, a short two-hour flight to Italy around Christmas. It was too hot to wear the stockings and I spent the whole flight feeling headachy and paranoid, worried I was critically endangering myself. I'm never able to relax on a flight anymore, no matter how long or short the distance.

In any case, while I survived that flight to Italy, I ended up with a worse problem on that trip. Just after Christmas, I was staying with some nuns in a convent in Perugia (which is another story), and likely as a result of whatever food they gave me – veganism not being widely understood in such parts – I probably ingested some egg pasta and possibly even dairy.

On 26 December, I was out walking a mile and a half from the convent when I got a horrible, crippling abdominal attack, similar to what had put me back in hospital again a few months earlier. I tried not to panic as I embarked on an extremely long and painful walk back to the convent, where thankfully I had a nice quiet room where I could rest and spend the remainder of the day. But I was very upset and anxious, and was on the phone to Trevor in tears, wondering if this was going to be my life from now on – plagued by sudden attacks in random places, sometimes far from home – and would I ever be free of this experience?

Psychological effects

Another consequence of my illness was that I lost a lot of self-confidence in my abilities. I had suffered a terrible ordeal, lost all of the strength in my muscles, got tired easily, had recurring stomach problems and was afraid of what to eat. I often had trouble concentrating and had immense difficulties processing anxiety, and was now no longer sure what I could put myself forward for.

Could I work for long periods of time? Could I volunteer in Italy, or further afield, as I had been planning to? What would I say to my host in the midst of a task – sorry but I have to rest now for two hours? I did eventually get to Italy at Christmas, as mentioned, and though the trip was full of hardships, including contracting a cold and the abdominal blockage described above, it did show me that I could rise to challenges and overcome difficulties, and that I still had some of the spark and initiative that I'd had before all of this happened.

However, I am no longer sure what I can do anymore, nor what I am capable of physically and emotionally. I look back to times when I was stronger and more fearless, but they're now interrupted by this great chasm of illness, showing me just how weak and debilitated I can become. Never mind how quickly I recovered – against all odds, and with everyone having had such negative views of the rate of my recovery. But it doesn't seem enough to me. Instead of considering how well I recovered, I see how quickly and thoroughly I fell into weakness, unable to do anything at all.

Sometimes now, when I'm tucking into a good meal, I remember how hard and depressing it was to eat anything, and what a relief it was when the 'meal' was over, even though I was still hungry. In that respect, and in aspects like walking, I marvel what a long way I've come, but it's never far from my mind just how low down it is possible to sink.

I suppose one of the hardest things to accept is being defined by this experience. Prior to this, I had never been seriously ill or stayed overnight in a hospital before. Apart from the laparoscopy day surgery I had undergone in 2010, I kept well away from hospitals where possible. Given my affinity with holistic healing, conventional medicine and hospitals were like foreign countries to me. In fact, a foreign country would have felt far more familiar. I certainly wouldn't have known anything about surgical procedures or critical care. I definitely knew nothing about bacterial infections, antibiotics or ICU equipment, compared to the extreme detail that I do now.

But, having been to hell and back, I can never ignore this experience. It's like it's drawn a line in my life, and I think about how I was before and how I've been since. It has marked me both physically and psychologically. Over a year later, many people still ask me how I am and remark on 'how well I look', more in reference to someone who has been critically ill than any other objective criteria. Some approach me with a newfound tenderness, bordering on pity, which I struggle not to rebuff.

But equally, it's also bred a kind of secrecy. There are people who know about what happened to me and people who don't, and it has defined who is in my life in a meaningful way. Trevor and I have become incredibly close as a result of this experience, particularly as there are many aspects which were only shared between us. With most new people I meet now, I'm reluctant to ever mention what happened to me, and usually do so only in passing, though it's always on the edge of my consciousness. I want to be the person I was before, and don't want new people to evaluate me based on someone who's been through such an extreme ordeal. Naturally, writing the book has been a big part of my recent life, and I often mention to people about having written it, though I try to focus on the more positive facets of the experience.

Writing the book has also helped a great deal with my coming to terms with what actually happened. Of course, it's very hard to process a traumatic experience, but it's so much harder when, for a large proportion of it, I wasn't actually present cognizantly, being delirious or unconscious during the worst stages of the disease. I now understand about delirium and know how common it is among patients in intensive care, and how the patient is absolutely convinced, as I was, that the imaginary world is what is actually going on. I have since been told repeatedly and in great detail about the things that truly did occur, but on some level they will never be real to me because I didn't actually experience them in any meaningful way. I've also come to appreciate very deeply how vital it was that there was someone present the whole time taking notes and compiling a diary of exactly what happened and when. Without Trevor's assiduous record keeping, the whole ICU experience would be one big haze, supplemented by memories of my fantasy world.

Sometimes I have very dark days, when I torture myself for having agreed to undergo the hysteroscopy in the first place. Writing this book has led me to do additional research, and I now know that my risks of contracting any kind of womb-related cancer were probably very slim. I only went through the procedure because I thought it would be a routine method of eliminating this remote possibility. Instead, as a result of taking what I thought was a precautionary measure, I lost an entire year of my life, have a weakened immune and digestive system, several ugly scars, lost my hair and generally do not feel like myself anymore. Another main area of torment is that, given that the procedure was meant to be so routine, why on earth were the results so catastrophic?

Inquiry

Even before I was discharged from hospital, I was burning with a passion to understand how a straightforward, diagnostic procedure ended up nearly killing me. I certainly left the hospital very confused about the whole situation and needing answers. Was there some degree of negligence involved?

Were there issues which had been brushed aside? In short, how could this possibly have happened?

While in hospital, I was assured that there would be an opportunity at a later stage for everything to be discussed with regards to my case. This, however, does not happen as a matter of course, but as a result of a formal procedure that must be instigated by the patient, who contacts the respective NHS trust and requests what's termed a 'local resolution meeting'. This involves all of the relevant medical parties meeting together to discuss the particular incident. As I set these wheels in motion immediately – two days after I was discharged, to be precise – I was fortunate to be granted a date for the meeting towards the end of the following month. This would be attended by Mr Ellis, Sandra and a couple of administrative hospital staff.

In the meantime, following the guidance of one of the doctors, I applied, and for a reasonable fee, obtained a copy of my medical records – 506 pages of photocopied details of all of my treatment. Obtaining medical records is a relatively straightforward process, which I highly recommend pursuing, as the notes have proven invaluable in clarifying exactly what procedures happened when and all the various medication I was given at different times.

The main purpose of the local resolution meeting was to discuss in detail with the consultants what had occurred, and to provide any likely explanations. It had already been established that the probable cause of the infection was that the hysteroscopy procedure, which involves using pressurised water, pushed bacteria from my urogenital tract into my body cavity, causing an infection which quickly escalated into septic shock. So Trevor and I had questions about the safety of the procedure, and why checks weren't made beforehand if there was the possibility of such a dangerous infection being spread.

We also wondered if this might have been considered grounds for legal action. The main issue for me wasn't so much one of liability as that of compensation. In effect, I had lost two months of being able to work and, without the help of my mum, would have been in great financial difficulty. Unfortunately, we discovered that the only way to obtain any kind of compensation was to go through the long and protracted legal process of suing the relevant NHS trust through a clinical negligence claim.

I looked into this to some considerable degree, contacting various law firms and obtaining initial advice, fortunately free of charge. The bottom line was that I had to be able to prove that either the procedure itself or the treatment of the resultant infection was carried out in a negligent way, and also that the procedure resulted in me suffering long-term damage that could otherwise have been avoided.

Though Trev and I had questions about the logic and safety of the procedure, we couldn't claim that it was carried out in a negligent way, nor could we fault how the infection was treated. Once sepsis was diagnosed, reaction times were swift and the appropriate treatment was rendered. What essentially kept me in the ICU so long was that the strain of infection I had was resistant to most antibiotics. I also did not incur any serious long-term damage directly as a result of the procedure. In short, our case was pretty flimsy, and at any rate, even before the inquiry, I had already decided not to pursue any legal action.

Compensation issues aside, at the end of the day, these doctors – whether they had put me in that state or not – did save my life, and I was reluctant to drag any of their names through the mud or point accusatory fingers. Also, a lawsuit such as this could potentially go on for years and incur crippling legal costs. Apparently, medical negligence claims are notoriously difficult to fight. Did I really want years of my life to be tied up in such a protracted battle?

Our main objective was to understand more fully how such a routine procedure resulted in such a life-threatening outcome. For us, it raised questions about the safety of the method involved. Since the hysteroscopy procedure involves forcing water from the urogenital tract to the abdominal cavity, it has the potential, as occurred with me, of spreading harmful bacteria, such as E. coli, into an area where it can become a life-threatening infection. Perhaps, we thought, some precautionary measures could be undertaken, such as a preventative medication or antibiotic to reduce the risk of spreading any agents of infection.

Both Ellis and Sandra's arguments were that, from the prior examinations undertaken, there was no evidence of a pre-existing infection, and that in a hysteroscopy, without the presence of such an infection, they would not give an antibiotic, so as not to overuse them and decrease their effectiveness.

Furthermore, the risks of anything major going awry from such a procedure are extremely low, with the escalation into sepsis virtually unheard of. Statistically, as outlined in the NHS hospital literature, serious complications arising from a diagnostic hysteroscopy are 2 women in every 1,000, while death occurs in 3–8 women in every 100,000. In my situation, the fact that these risks were dealt with in a perfunctory way, as in the pre-surgery consent form, is meant to be indicative of how rare such a disastrous outcome is. This proved to be a major theme of the local resolution meeting.

However, we still felt that even with the stated risks being statistically so low, if the potential outcome of a pathogen being spread can have such serious consequences, then perhaps the way the procedure is carried out should at least be considered.

We attempted – and failed – to have the experience listed as what's termed a 'serious untoward incident', which would have necessitated a resultant 'root cause analysis' investigation, but it was determined that as the risks of it occurring again were so slight, that this was not an avenue deemed worth pursuing.

Instead, the incident was downgraded to 'negligible' because the impact of the incident was negligible on the efficacy of the health services, being that it was a rare, extreme complication of the procedure. Or, as Ellis put it, 'The magnitude is massive for you, but when we look at it more broadly across the population, because the incidence is so low, there isn't felt to be the need to change what's happening.'

Trev and I emerged from the inquiry both confused and deflated. We came away without any satisfactory explanation as to why, given that the procedure entails the enforced movement of potentially harmful bacteria into an area ill-equipped to combat its effects, what happened to me doesn't occur more often. Or, to put it the reverse way around, if this generally doesn't ever occur amongst the general population, then why *did* it happen to me? The consultants threw their hands up and declared that some things that happened in medicine were simply a mystery.

We also got the feeling that the well-established medics were keen to put this exceedingly irregular incident summarily behind them. There were some noises made about the case being used anonymously in lectures, as a rare example of how the procedure can very occasionally result in extreme consequences.

There was also talk of how lessons could be learned in the effectiveness of interventional radiology in similar circumstances, and on the possibility of reducing the recommended course of rivaroxaban for treating a DVT, but that was about it. We left the inquiry with the gnawing sense that, despite all of our efforts, this whole episode was effectively going to be filed away and forgotten.

Lessons learned

Instead, it made me feel that the best way forward was to try and contribute towards raising awareness about sepsis and its potential outcomes, as well as the options available as an NHS patient. I think it's important to note that from what I've been hearing from other sepsis survivors, there is very little aftercare offered by hospitals, especially by way of counselling or support, which many patients or relatives strongly need to process their trauma and confusion.

There are attempts to bridge this gap by groups like the UK Sepsis Trust, a small but very dedicated charitable organisation which supports both survivors and those bereaved by a loved one lost to sepsis, as well as raising awareness about its symptoms. I stumbled upon the organisation in a local newspaper, and indeed, the group says they are now getting increased media coverage, while nationally, throughout health care sectors, there are growing numbers of campaigns being conducted to improve both the diagnosis and treatment of sepsis.

There is still much that is not properly understood about sepsis. One of its more challenging aspects is that the illness can be contracted in a myriad of ways, ranging from cold symptoms to post-operative complications, and the tell-tale indicators are not always immediately clear. Sepsis can develop from an infection anywhere in the body, and while the elderly and those with weakened immune systems are more at risk, anyone can develop sepsis, including the young and healthy.

As medical recording becomes more accurate, reported incidents of sepsis are increasing. Currently in the UK, over 100,000 people a year suffer from sepsis, out of which over 30% die as a result, while a quarter of survivors suffer life-altering disabilities, such as organ dysfunction or limb amputations. I consider myself to be one of the lucky ones, despite the unlikely way in which it happened to me. I've added my story to the UK Sepsis Trust website and intend to utilise aspects of my story, such as this book, as a way of helping others understand and move on from their own experiences.

One of the chief aspects I'm raising awareness about is making informed decisions with regards to one's own healing, and to have the courage to do so in the face of an established authority. It's often impossible to predict if a procedure will result in complications or to control the way in which it is carried out. However, I can strongly encourage people to take charge of their recovery process, wherever possible. It is an important message for me to impart, that one has rights and choices in hospital about the treatments received, and that, even when feeling at your most vulnerable, it's important not to accept blindly whatever is being offered.

Instead, it is imperative to take ownership of your recovery options and – with the help and support of family and friends, where possible – to try and work in partnership with the medical staff to make rational, intuitive decisions that are right for you, and feel confident that they will be willing to listen. This was my experience, and I was very fortunate that, as the NHS advocates patient-centred medicine, the medical team were willing to work in tandem with Trevor and myself. It was admirable how much they respected our individual wishes and views, and were especially accommodating with regards to allowing us to meet all of my food and nutritional requirements in our own way.

Similarly, there were medical procedures we disagreed with and resisted, such as the tracheotomy and the full pelvic clearance surgery, and we were able to reason our way to arrive at better solutions. Indeed, it was Trevor's faith in the effectiveness of the radiological drainage procedure – even in the face of the doctors' doubts – that allowed it to go ahead, and it was this expertly performed procedure which turned the corner in my road to recovery. As such, I've learned that in any medical situation, no matter how serious or absolute it appears to be, it is always worth discussing and putting forward your concerns or points of view if you feel strongly that what you're being offered is not right for you.

A hospital, like any other organisation, operates with its own established rules and regulations. No matter how kind and attentive the individual nurses and medical team were, it was still standardised, procedural care. As in many workplaces, it's easy to become institutionalised, and to get used to a basic set of rules and to begin to think that it's normal. I know certainly when I was in hospital one of the things that disturbed me most was how easily I got used to and accepted what was a very odd day-to-day routine. But even within a set framework, it's extremely important never to lose your integrity or sense of what you think and feel is right.

As excellent as the hospital team were, I've learned how much of healing is down to the individual. From practically the time I emerged from a coma, I didn't know what I was doing in intensive care, but I knew instinctively that I should not continue to be there, and would not get better if I remained there under constant scrutiny. I truly believe that alongside the effective medical treatment, it was the communication with my body and my will to get better that accelerated my healing.

The medical profession ascribes healing solely to whatever treatment is being administered. The positive attitude or motivation of the individual is not necessarily considered. Medically, there is a measurement for everything but there is no measurement for personal will, or for the light that radiates from within. I consider my will and steadfast determination to return to health to account for at least half of the reason that I recovered – and so quickly.

For many sepsis survivors, it can sometimes take up to eighteen months before they can feel back to how they were before. For me, although I do still get tired and have my bad days, overall, I've since led a fairly active life. I went to Italy three months later on my own and, after working in admin for a year and saving up, have planned a bigger trip to Australia. So, something other than medical science must account for my ability to have recovered so rapidly and completely.

Like most things in life, the experience is what you make of it. Surviving sepsis can make you feel like an unlucky victim, and be debilitating both physically and psychologically. But equally, by trying to extract something positive from the experience, surviving such a life-threatening infection can be a means of empowering your life for the future.

As such, over time, I've tried to become more philosophical about the whole experience. Indeed, it is always preferable to think that things happen for a reason. Surviving sepsis has provided me with knowledge about all kinds of things I never thought I would have, especially not at my age or state of good health. And, apart from my very strong need for something positive to emerge from this experience, I sincerely hope that the lessons I've learned can be passed on to others, and that people who have suffered from sepsis or from some other kind of serious illness will feel less helpless or alone. It has made me want to share what happened to me with others, in the hope that people can learn to empower themselves too, even in the most dire and hopeless-looking situations.

The experience has also taught me about what real love and devotion is, and how incredible it is to have someone by your side, fighting your corner and caring for you in a deep, compassionate and meaningful way. Indeed, for me, love, dedication and compassion are the driving factors of all life.

A consultant recently said to me that it's up to me how much store I put on this experience, and that I can identify with it as much or as little as I want. If I had just broken my arm or was in hospital for some other reason I could possibly agree. But surviving a near-death experience can't help but become part of your life and how you view things, and inform what is important, and how many things are not. While I try to exercise compassion, I find I am often now quite impatient with people who obsess over what seem to me to be very petty matters.

It has also made me less willing to be involved with things that are wrong for me, including various avenues of work, as I've realised how precious life is, and that it can't be squandered doing things that are not healthy for me, particularly spiritually. In that respect, I've become less lazy in my thinking and actions and am getting better at pursuing options that feel right, no matter how illogical they may seem on paper.

Certainly, while I was in hospital I didn't think, 'Oh I can't wait to get home and do nothing.' The first day I woke up in Hawthorn Ward, I saw the birds outside on the tree, and had the epiphany that I had to get better because I wanted to help make a difference in the world, especially to wildlife, and that I needed to get on with my plans in a very pressing way.

In fact, I still feel this way, but the reality of getting things going is often more difficult than the idea and takes so much longer. This has been one of the hardest aspects of recovery. I thought as soon as I made it home I would be setting my new plans into motion. Many days I get discouraged and depressed about how little things seem to have changed, when I feel like I should have been catapulted into my new, energised and meaningful life. I guess healing itself is a longer process, and I need to exercise a certain degree of patience while I build up my strength and work with the powers that be towards furthering my aims.

The experience of going in for a routine procedure and emerging nearly dead has also taught me that there are absolutely no securities in life. But the real danger is being too afraid to live life authentically, to let fear keep you from achieving your dreams. One of the clearest messages I got from the universe is if I can survive that experience, then I'm capable of achieving anything – including writing a book about it all!

In any case, what is the worst that can happen? Having already experienced the worst – the finality of death – this has made me realise that it is never too late to try and try again, and to learn from one's continuing attempts. 'Where there is life, there is hope' is my new maxim, and it is always, *always* – whatever the circumstances – worth following and pursuing your dreams.

I feel this intensely because I've learned – at a very visceral level – just how fragile life is and how quickly and readily it can be taken away. Everyone knows this on some intellectual level, but to experience it so profoundly – how easily it can happen for no apparent or anticipated reason – has to change one's view towards life and intensify the urgency of getting on with things.

Life is too precious to waste even a single second of it. We all get sucked into the minutiae of our lives without realising that a life not lived to its full potential is a terrible waste, and how quickly it can be taken away without warning. The universe is not going to wait while you say, 'Maybe I'll do it next year.' There simply may not be a next year.

Life has to be seized with both hands, and lived fully and immediately. We have a duty to ourselves to fulfil our potential and be the best person we can be. The real crime in life is not when or how we die, but if we have never really lived.

POSTSCRIPT

On the up Down Under

January 2017

I was only going to write a paragraph or two on my time in Australia (and New Zealand), only to say that I made the journey and returned again in one piece. But I learned so much on this trip – about Australia, yes, but so much more about my own abilities in facing challenges, and the repositories of strength I found to draw upon to propel me forward and to try new things. Truly, I had many awe-inspiring experiences, undertook deeply fulfilling volunteer opportunities and had wondrous encounters with beautiful wildlife. But for me, the real triumph of the journey was how much it enabled me to grow and become a stronger, more resolute and fuller individual.

This was an enormous trip to be taking alone, and while Trevor supported my journey completely, he did not wish to accompany me on this extended foray halfway around the world. So it would be fair to say that I embarked on this massive expedition with a reasonable amount of trepidation. Apart from personal, family-related issues obscuring my preparations, I certainly did not feel 100 per cent well by the time I left – just over a year after I had contracted sepsis – and I was still having stomach problems, especially in the mornings. How was it going to be when I wasn't in control of what and when I could eat? What if I got another small bowel blockage? Would I need to be rushed to hospital? And how much energy was I going to have to do anything in general, let alone volunteering? What about getting a blood clot from the long flights? The list of worries went on and on. But still I went.

All these issues (and more) remained ever-present throughout my entire trip. I'd like to say that all my health concerns magically disappeared, being on an extended holiday away from everyday stresses, but my stomach problems persisted all the way through the three-month sojourn (though I'm happy to say a couple of skin conditions cleared up thanks to the drier, warmer climate).

In any event, it simply became a case of dealing with issues as and when they arose. I learned to avoid a lot of foods (*a lot* of foods) and deal with the problems in whatever way I had to. Eating was always a challenge and one I never got completely right, and I was often hungry and tired, trying to avoid all the foods that could potentially trigger a reaction.

Fortunately, Australia, especially in the bigger cities, is pretty good for veganism and gluten-free options (which I was experimenting with), so I found many staples I could eat daily, like rice crackers and almonds. However, sometimes limited choices and being on the road so much meant I ended up not eating as well as I would have liked. But Australia is very good at providing water fountains, clean public loos and parks where I could have a nap if I needed one. It also helped that the majority of people I met throughout my travels were very easy going, understanding and kind.

Mercifully, in the three months I was there I only had a small bowel blockage problem once, which, admittedly, was pretty awful. I think it was most likely triggered by a highly processed cereal given to me for breakfast at a place I was staying at, in New Zealand. The pain was pretty ferocious and, as it hit while I was out (and quite far from the accommodation), the only thing I could do was make my way slowly to the nearest park I could find – which turned out to be the grounds of a church – and lie down on the grass, with a lawnmower roaring and people regularly passing by. I had to lie completely still for an hour before I felt well enough to get up again, and even then I had to tread very lightly the rest of the day. But thankfully the pain passed, and with it the scariest health problem of the entire trip.

In second place was when I thought I had developed a blood clot, as a searing pain reappeared in the exact spot on my left ankle where the original clot had been. I was used to odd pains appearing in my legs (especially since I had fallen quite badly and bruised my legs some weeks before). But it was the fact that the pain was in the same place as the original clot, combined with me having been on a three-hour flight a few days before (without wearing the embolic stockings) that caused me so much worry. I considered going to the medical clinic I noticed in town, but in the meantime, I did what seemed to work with all my other pains – I remained aware of it and hoped it would go away in time. It was unfortunate that it occurred in the few days I was hiking in the Blue Mountains near Sydney – the sometimes vertical terrain a challenge at the best of times.

But there was nothing I could do if I wanted to enjoy the spectacular scenery, except to go slowly and avoid putting too much pressure on my left foot as I juddered up and down the steep, winding steps into the valleys. It took a long time and was pretty painful, but the ethereal surroundings made it well worth it in the end. And thankfully, the pain in my ankle – which I later discovered may well have been a blood clot – went away in a few days, as mysteriously as it had appeared.

But such misfortunes were made up for by the sheer awesomeness of the experiences I was having: redesigning tourist brochures in a historic town in New South Wales, visiting a sanctuary for orphaned joeys in the middle of the Outback, or way up in the mountains, waking up to kangaroos hopping outside my window. I couldn't ignore the problems, but the important thing was that I was dealing with them as they arose, and they weren't impeding my ability to remain active and engaged in my environment. To me, this active engagement is not only an essential part of healing, but is also vital for continuing to maintain one's overall health.

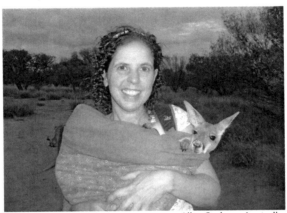

Pure joy. At a kangaroo sanctuary near Alice Springs, Australia.

There was one time I went on a guided wildlife walk in coastal New Zealand, and I huffed and puffed up a rocky incline. I later found out that the walk leader had divided the group into two routes – a tough one and an easier one, for those who he thought couldn't cope with the terrain. Being Canadian, and therefore deemed to be hardier, the guide opted to put me on the tougher route – if he only knew!

But the journey taught me what I was truly capable of. Every decision I had to make myself, and every problem I had to solve alone, as there was literally no one to do it for me. I wasn't able to ruminate on how to get somewhere or where to find food I could safely eat. Instead, I just had to do it and figure it out as I went along, and put all my energies into the most effective way to get what I needed for that particular day.

I actually found this inability to prevaricate or procrastinate quite liberating, as I basically had to get on with things if I wanted to achieve anything on the trip. I'm not saying it was easy; it was often quite difficult and lonely. Thankfully, Trevor was on hand (via Skype) to act as a pressure release, but really, it was up to me. So instead, I found myself adopting the 'in for a penny, in for a pound' maxim and undertook experiences well beyond my regular comfort zone, such as hiking and snorkelling solo, or sleeping under the stars in a swag.

This constantly challenging myself and being rewarded by my efforts made me realise that with motivation, one is truly capable of achieving anything. Getting well again was one thing, but this extended trip, with its myriad of challenges, proved that with determination, I could genuinely accomplish anything I put my mind and heart into. And I truly believe this is possible for anyone.

In this respect, I now feel that in some ways I was a lot *more* unwell before the whole sepsis episode, because I was often so self-defeating and disinterested in life. Maybe now I have some lasting physical impediments that I didn't before, but the insights I've gained in valuing and appreciating life – in acting on what feels right and staying motivated and engaged, wherever it may take me – all of this has made me a better, stronger, person, and overall I feel *more well* than I ever did before. There is an equivalent of an Australian trip – or whatever your passion may be – waiting inside all of us. I hope that you too will have the strength and courage to learn to live up to your fullest potential.